BEYOND THE TAPE

The Life and Many Deaths of
a State Pathologist

Professor Marie Cassidy became a forensic pathologist in 1985 following her training as a histopathologist.

She worked as a consultant forensic pathologist in the Department of Forensic Medicine and Toxicology in Glasgow for the next thirteen years investigating unnatural deaths and homicides, from gangland shootings and stabbings, to drug deaths, road traffic accidents and suicides.

In 1998 she returned to her family's homeland of Ireland as deputy state pathologist, working alongside Professor Jack Harbison. When he retired, she was appointed state pathologist and, like her predecessor, her name became synonymous with murder and tragedy. In over thirty years of practice she has performed thousands of postmortems and dealt with hundreds of murders.

Marie retired at the end of 2018 and now lives in London. *Beyond the Tape* is her first book.

BEYOND THE TAPE

The Life and Many Deaths
of a State Pathologist

DR. MARIE CASSIDY

HACHETTE
BOOKS
IRELAND

First published in Ireland in 2021 by Hachette Books Ireland
First published in paperback in 2021

Cataloguing in Publication Data is available from the British Library

ISBN 978 1 52935 260 3

Typeset in Sabon by redrattledesign.com
Printed and bound in Great Britain by Clays Ltd, Elcograf S.p.A.

The author and publishers would like to thank the following: Gwen Malone
Stenography Services, for permission to reproduce court transcripts in the book;
The Stunning, for permission to reproduce lyrics from 'This Happy Girl'; the
Pellenz family, the Murphy family, Paul Maxwell Photography, Joe Cashin, Brian
Lawless/PA Images, Collins Agency, True Media Photography and Ann Power, for
permission to reproduce images.

Hachette Books Ireland policy is to use papers that are natural, renewable
and recyclable products and made from wood grown in sustainable forests.
The logging and manufacturing processes are expected to conform to the
environmental regulations of the country of origin.

Hachette Books Ireland
8 Castlecourt Centre
Castleknock
Dublin 15, Ireland

A division of Hachette UK Ltd
Carmelite House, 50 Victoria Embankment, EC4Y 0DZ

www.hachettebooksireland.ie

To my family. This might explain all those times I wasn't there. Sorry.

'Justice cannot be for one side alone, but must be for both.'
Eleanor Roosevelt

Contents

Pre-mortem

'GUILTY OF MURDER', 'NOT GUILTY of murder but guilty of manslaughter', 'Not guilty' and, in Scotland, 'Not proven'. That's how murder trials end. But where do they begin and how do we get to the end result? Well, I'm part of the process of investigating murders – emphasis on the *r* as I'm Scottish: I'm a forensic pathologist. Not that I always admit it. In the early days no one knew what a forensic pathologist was but now, thanks to the power of the media, everyone seems to think they're an expert in all things forensic. All hail *CSI*.

In fact, very few television programmes represent the role of the forensic pathologist accurately. Their forensic pathologist tends to be part pathologist, part police, part forensic scientist. Trust me, it is nowhere near as interesting or glamorous as TV makes it look.

Taggart was probably most accurate in its portrayal, as the pathologist was confined to the mortuary and, once the postmortem was over, that was the end of their role. A bit part but essential to establish that *Taggart* was dealing with murder. Even then, though, the programme was not entirely accurate as in Scotland, due to the legal requirement of corroboration of all relevant facts in a criminal case, two forensic pathologists are required to examine every potential murder. Probably due to budgetary concerns, only one pathologist was portrayed in the programme, the stereotypical middle-aged bearded male.

The only forensic pathologist I have ever met who personified the writer's assumption was John – or Jack as everyone knew him – Harbison, professor of forensic medicine and state pathologist in Ireland. At any forensic conference he was the stand-out 'poster boy' for the profession. As a concession to legal accuracy, when filming a mortuary scene in

Taggart there would be a lingering shot of an empty pair of wellingtons, implying a second pathologist without the expense. It was not until 2001 that a female forensic pathologist was introduced, some sixteen years after the first was appointed in Glasgow. Despite the fact that I had been a consultant to the programme for years.

When *Silent Witness* came along in 1996, the lead was a female forensic pathologist, reflecting the increasing numbers of women attracted to a career in the discipline. But they had to beef up the part, and suddenly the forensic pathologist was the key figure in murder investigations, not just one of the backroom boys or girls. Routinely Dr Sam Ryan was seen questioning witnesses – as if the police would ever let a pathologist near one.

Since then, there has been some confusion as to what forensic pathologists do. The answer is simple: we carry out postmortem examinations to establish the cause of death, even if it appears blatantly obvious in some cases, and in doing so identify deaths due to homicide. The whole system of death investigation was largely designed to prevent homicides going undetected, but now it is more encompassing and plays an important role in monitoring the health of the population. The role of the forensic pathologist has, however, remained true to the original ethos: was the death due to a murder, or not?

When people hear I am a forensic pathologist, the response is usually, 'How, or why, did you become a forensic pathologist?' followed by 'What was the worst/most gruesome case you were involved with?'

The 'how' is usually asked by schoolchildren or medical students with an interest in forensics, not necessarily forensic pathology, who wonder how easy it is to get into the world of *CSI*. The short answer to that is 'It's not easy.' The question 'why' is usually asked by medical colleagues. In Glasgow the implication was that I obviously wasn't good enough to be a 'hospital' pathologist (I was, and got my MRCPath on the first attempt), but in Ireland it was more a case of 'Are you off your bloody head? You could earn double and not be on call working late nights and weekends.' Fair point, but for me it's not about the money, although that does not entitle my paymasters to take advantage of my good nature.

As for the other question – the most gruesome case I've seen – it's usually male transition-year students or budding psychopaths who ask. I dodge that one as, sure as Fate, either Mammy would be on the phone claiming I'd traumatised her darling son, or the details would be on the front page of *The Sun* (it has happened).

This is my attempt to answer those questions more fully. Specifically to take the reader beyond the police tape and into the real world of forensic pathology, not the *Quincy* version (for those of a similar vintage to myself) or the *CSI/Silent Witness* version (for younger readers). I'll talk about the origins of forensic pathology, its modern-day practice, and my sometimes fascinating, sometimes heartrending journey through it, over more than three decades.

1

Beginning

THE PLANE LANDED IN SIERRA Leone in the summer of 2000. By UN standards it had been a relatively uneventful journey via Guinea. Robert McNeill, a senior anatomical pathology technician, manager of the mortuary in the Western Infirmary in Glasgow, and I were picked up by UN personnel and taken to a hotel on the beach in Freetown, the capital. The hotel had been taken over by the UN as their headquarters in 1999 when they assumed the role of peacekeepers following the civil war, which had been raging since the early 1990s.

Here we met the other members of the group. Our mission was to recover the bodies of a small group of UN soldiers, killed in the ongoing conflict. We were to identify the men and determine the cause of their death. We were told that it might be difficult to get to the site, but were reassured that the issue would be resolved in the next day or so. I was the forensic pathologist responsible for determining the cause of death and Robert had to secure mortuary facilities. I had travelled from Ireland and he had come from Glasgow, but we had worked together since the 1980s and were firm friends. Sue Black, a forensic anthropologist with a large, hugely successful university department in Dundee, was to join us. She and I had worked together on several cases when I was still in Glasgow.

She was responsible for identification. In addition, there was forensic radiographer Mark Viner, and scenes of crime officers (SOCOs), including a photographer, fingerprinter and exhibits curator, all from England, to assist in the recovery of the bodies, to record and photograph the findings. The Nigerian and Indian armies were responsible for our safety while we were in Sierra Leone.

The trench where the bodies lay was behind enemy lines, hence the difficulty with gaining access to them. We hoped that the UN Army would push the rebels back long enough for us to recover them. Suddenly it dawned on me that maybe my husband was right to be a bit annoyed at my cavalier attitude to my safety, and the repercussions on the family if it all went pear-shaped. Sue was informed by the British government that she was not to move from the hotel until they had been assured of her safety. Nobody seemed too concerned about myself, Robert or Mark so we were on standby, waiting for the signal that the enemy line had moved back and we had a short window of opportunity to get in and out.

The next morning we were picked up, put on a helicopter and taken into the 'jungle'. We were debriefed by the Nigerian commander, who said that we should move in as soon as we were given the signal but to keep our heads down: as Europeans, we were an easy target. A jeep took us deeper into the bush. Gunfire was raging. We sat for what seemed like hours until we were told that the enemy line had been pushed back although the UN Army couldn't predict how long they could keep the rebels contained. We ran across the ground to the trench, keeping our heads down. It took a few hours but eventually we had excavated the bodies and documented our findings. We had completed the first phase successfully, without any casualties.

At this point we were handed over to the Indian Army. We were told we were invited to lunch and off we went again in the jeep. A short drive away from enemy lines we came to a camp. We were expecting army rations served on tin plates and couldn't believe our eyes. In the clearing a magnificent tent rose out of the jungle, like a mini Taj Mahal. We were each offered a bowl of hot water to wash, then were served with the best Indian meal I had ever had, with wine in real glasses.

We returned to the hotel to update our colleagues and make arrangements for the postmortems the following day. Luckily the local hospital pathologist had agreed to make his mortuary available to us. The next morning we drove into Freetown to the hospital. Despite the obvious poverty, the people living in shacks, the majority seemed relatively happy, and the children were in school uniform, with blindingly white shirts and socks. There was evidence of the war, men badly scarred and many with missing limbs, but life was going on.

We reached the mortuary, which was a dark, dank room with the most basic facilities, but sufficient for our needs. It was claustrophobic and the stench was overpowering. The postmortems were relatively straightforward: we managed to identify the men and determine the cause of their deaths. At one point I went outside for a breath of fresh air. The mortuary was behind and set back from the hospital on an area of scrubland. I leaned against the door and had a look around. At the side of the building there was a tree, bare of leaves, and perched on the branches, two large vultures stared down at the mortuary entrance.

A shiver ran down my spine. How on earth did I end up here? I had never planned to be a forensic pathologist. Like most of the major events in my life, marriage, children, moving country, it had happened without much thought on my part. I was the middle child of three, and Dad was the local coalman. I'm sure most of his customers thought we had a charmed life and it seemed fine to me. We started out in a one-bedroom semi-detached council house in a little village called Craigneuk, about twenty miles from Glasgow, but when I was about seven we moved to a three-bedroom semi in Wishaw, a few miles up the road. There, my little sister Monica and I now had a room to ourselves and my brother Jim, seven years older than me, got his own room. We thought we were on the way up.

However, when we compared our lives to those of our friends there were some differences. On Friday nights and Saturdays we worked in the family business: we collected the 'tick money', the money owed for the coal delivered to the customers during the week. The job qualifications were fairly lenient: you just had to be able to count the cost of two bags of coal, a bag of dross and some firelighters, and calculate the change from a fiver. Once we were proficient at arithmetic we were on the payroll. Well, not exactly, but we had money to buy sweets at school the coming week. I was top of the class in arithmetic, particularly mental arithmetic.

So, from the age of six or seven Monica and I were 'helping out'. Sometimes we were taken round the customers' houses in the car but it was so much more fun in the lorry. As we were so small we had to leap ninja-style onto the footplate, then clamber into the cab, often while the lorry was moving along. Health and safety wasn't a consideration. I still remember where I was when we heard of John F. Kennedy's death: collecting coal money on the 'back road'. Dad wasn't very good with road names or towns, but we knew where he meant. He was even worse with people's names (must be genetic: I have the same problem). He took name association to a different level: Cats was a woman with more than a few (I tried to avoid going into her house while she found the money as the smell was pretty powerful) and Pinny was an older woman who had asked Dad to get her a new apron, or pinny, to wear to the 'Orange Walk' ('Even if you are a Catholic, Mr Cassidy') as she couldn't get to the shops. He was very obliging.

Life would have continued as 'normal', had Dad avoided what they called in those days 'hardening of the arteries', atherosclerosis, caused partly by genetic hyper-cholesterolaemia (I've got that too) but mostly by an unhealthy smoking habit of eighty-plus cigarettes a day (I avoided that). I only knew that he couldn't take us out for a walk as he had to stop every few minutes because of pain in his legs, a condition known as intermittent claudication. This necessitated surgery and many stints in hospital. His business suffered but I was delighted to be getting home earlier on Friday nights and Saturday afternoons because we didn't have so many customers. It was then that the early seeds of a career in medicine must have been sown: I spent most Sundays visiting Dad and other poorly relatives in hospital. My weekends were well and truly scuppered, working Friday night and Saturday, mass on Sunday morning and hospital Sunday afternoon. Where are social services when you need them?

Anyway, school progressed well, still top of the class for arithmetic, and at eleven I was off to secondary school where, as happened in those days, I was streamed into the sciences rather than languages, which suited me fine. I loved physics. Mr Duffy, the physics teacher, really did make it fun. My five years at Bothwell, Elmwood Senior Secondary, were mostly good but I must confess that I wasn't that fond of school, I think it was the children. I've never been a big fan of children, even when I was one. I was looking forward to finishing but, having been 'working' for the last nine or ten years, I wasn't that keen on leaving school to get a job in a bank like some of my friends.

During that time Dad had several heart attacks and, despite the operations on the leg arteries, he ended up having one limb amputated. He tried to continue working but that would have meant us helping him in and out of the lorry, which wasn't feasible long term. This probably shaped my future: when I was asked to choose which subject I would study if I went to university, I said, 'Medicine,' much to the consternation of the nuns. They thought us girls should be nuns, teachers, nurses, or wives and mothers. I was amazed myself, but once it was out, there was no going back. I went home and told Dad, who was now bedbound, and he was delighted. Just a few months later he had a stroke and died. I had to follow through now.

I haven't mentioned my mum. She was Scarlett O'Hara to his Rhett Butler. He scrubbed up well, she was glamorous and fun-loving, and tomorrow was just another day. Life must have taken a very different turn from what she'd expected when she married the only eligible bachelor in the village. As Dad's health declined she had to step up to the mark. A life of comparative leisure was replaced by taking the helm in a dirty business, which included going out in the lorry to make sure money kept coming in. God knows what her hairdresser thought of the normally blonde curls now flecked with coal dust. Eventually even she had to admit that she couldn't cope: the business folded, and suddenly I had my weekends back.

A few weeks after Dad died I was doing my

exams to get into university. Luckily I got the results required for medicine and I was accepted by Glasgow University. At seventeen I was on the road to a medical degree. As usual I didn't think much about the money situation. In Scotland, coming from a single-parent family (Mum was now working as an insurance agent, which meant I still had to collect money on a Saturday) I was eligible for a grant to cover tuition fees, travel and living expenses. Despite our reduced circumstances, there was still a supposed parental contribution, which Mum interpreted as me contributing to my parent, so I was back to working on a Friday night as well as a Saturday in a local bar and restaurant in order to have money for train fares and any kind of social life.

University was an education in all senses. Suddenly from being regarded as pretty intelligent, in the top 10 per cent of the school, you find you're average in comparison to the others. No longer do you look at exam results from the top down but from the bottom up, only taking a breath when you get over the 50 per cent.

My introduction to anything like a patient came during my second year, in anatomy. In 1972, thanks to people generously donating their bodies, medical students were taught anatomy by the meticulous dissection of the human body. Generally, anatomy departments are dark buildings, with the pervasive sickly smell of embalming fluids. About eight of us were to work on an adult male. We were given no details as to who he had been or even how he died. Now I know that the identities are kept secret and the bodies are carefully selected to try to ensure that the students are not confused by variations in anatomy, whether natural or due to surgery. The authorities are very picky about who they accept. Thankfully, by the time the selection process is in full swing, the donor is unaware of the goings-on and won't be upset if they're turned down for full dissection because they're obese, had too many surgeries or are just surplus to requirements. Nevertheless, cornea can still be harvested and other parts used for research.

Our body had a tattoo, a heart with the name Bessie, so he became known affectionately as Bessie's boyfriend. I like to think that over the course of the year we learned more about him than Bessie ever did. Which reminds me: tattoos are useful for identification purposes but if you have recorded the names of your paramours, current and ex, in glorious technicolour across your body, you might want to consider a line through the defunct ones, just in case.

Medical schools should perhaps monitor the anatomy sessions closely as at this point the personality traits that will determine which branch of medicine you might be most suited to become apparent. I wanted to do the dissection slowly and carefully but, as the smallest and youngest, I was pushed out by the more forceful members of the group, some of whom wanted to spend as little time as possible in the dissection room. As a result of their overenthusiastic work, some parts of the body are still a trifle hazy to me. But even I didn't want to spend too much time on each and every bone in the hands and feet. Thank God for anthropologists. However, it didn't make much difference to the time spent as to whether or not you stank of formalin. But it did clear a room, useful if you were trying to get a drink at the always crowded student bars, which by now I was old enough to frequent. At any rate anatomy had got me thinking.

Once we had the nuts and bolts under our belts it was time to introduce us to living patients. This was when it started to go wrong. By now we were two years down, four to go. Perhaps a more integrated approach, introducing patients at the start, would make it easier for students to switch course if they thought it might not be for them. I began with renal dialysis. Should be easy: generally healthy people, delighted to have company to dispel the boredom of waiting for toxins to be filtered from their blood. That's what did it for me: blood in tubes running between man and machine. I woke up on the bed next to the nice man I had been chatting to.

Next was the operating theatre. The procedure was a haemorrhoidectomy. The floor was a bit harder to land on. If nothing else, I was beginning to know what branch of medicine I wasn't best suited to. For the next four years I crossed specialities off the list with increasing rapidity. Pregnant women and babies? No. Children? Even the consultant said, 'No.' Anything to do with working in a ward that might entail wandering around a hospital in the middle of the night was also a no. I reached that decision following a stint as a locum in a surgical ward. In those days medical students were required to cover for interns who were on holiday. I remember standing at the window of the surgical ward at two o'clock one morning, thinking, What am I doing here in charge of all these sick people?

I was reaching the end of my training without any idea of what I was going to do. Within six months I would be a doctor. The medical profession had invested six years in me and wanted me to succeed. I had only ever failed one exam, in public health, but in my defence they were asking about obstetrics and gynaecology somewhere in Africa, and I'd had enough trouble with 'obs and gynae' in Glasgow. I had to re-sit, which gave me six months' breathing space.

Instead of starting as an intern I went on holiday for a month and returned much happier as I now had a plan: pathology. No live patients, only little pieces in a jar, and postmortem examinations. Now I could finish my degree, get through my internship and my career would be on track.

My internship confirmed my decision to leave patients behind: it was hard to reconcile six-plus years of study to end up filing blood test results. However, as I was working in peripheral hospitals, I often found myself, the most junior doctor in the hospital, being 'it' at nights and weekends. It was a wonder anyone left the hospital alive. The hours we worked were preposterous. Our average week was three twelve-hour day shifts, an extended shift to midnight and an overnighter. Then we were on call one weekend in three, which dropped to one in two when someone went off sick.

The weekend on call started Friday morning and ended Monday morning. Occasionally a senior doctor, nicely rested after their weekend golfing or whatever, would take pity on you and let you go early after the Monday-morning ward round, but only after you'd taken bloods and followed up results on tests you might have ordered. Sometimes we were asked to do minor procedures that we were unfamiliar with but were in the interns' handbook. On one occasion an old gentleman asked Sister if he could have his ears syringed before he was discharged that afternoon. The handbook didn't stipulate that it was best to use warm water as cold water in the ear tends to cause the eyes to flick back and forth rapidly, rendering the patient nauseous and dizzy. But at least he heard my apology. The test I had carried out, cold water in the ear, is now routinely used to determine that someone is brain dead. My old gentleman was definitely alive.

I spent a year as a nomad, trekking from ward to ward, speciality to speciality. My one mistake, which I was aware of, was forgetting to prescribe penicillin for a patient coming out of theatre one

Friday night. Normally a hanging offence. The mistake was noticed the next morning during the ward round. As the consultant vented his spleen about the inadequacies of the intern (me) the patient piped up that he had forgotten to mention he was allergic to penicillin. The consultant turned on the patient. I had to apologise to both consultant and patient for my mistake. I didn't mention that I had inadvertently saved the patient's life. But I always learn from my mistakes. Always check if people have allergies. Always make sure you follow instructions.

I very nearly veered off course when I ended up doing a stint in Accident and Emergency. It really was just like the telly. People coming in fast and furious. Head pains, road traffic accidents, broken arms and legs, nose bleeds, mental health issues, a plethora of complaints. Part of the beauty was that you treated them and they went off, usually never to be seen again. This was a hospital in the sticks so there weren't specialists on hand: I was expected to be a plastic surgeon, stitching the faces of those who had exited a moving car through the windscreen, an ENT specialist, packing bleeding noses and syringing ears (remembering to use warm water), and even an ophthalmologist picking foreign bodies out of eyes. None of that would be allowed now without proper training, and it really shouldn't have been then.

Another duty was putting plaster casts on fractured limbs. The 'plasterers' didn't work nights or weekends, and this was yet another skill we were not taught at medical school. It appeared to be the old adage, if someone with one O level (UK) or Junior Cert (Ireland) could do it, surely someone with a medical degree could. Have you ever tried wallpapering? Enough said. Luckily all patients with fractures had to see an orthopaedic surgeon the next day in case they needed surgical fixation. Having made the diagnosis of a fracture, all I had to do was make sure things didn't get any worse for twenty-four hours. My remedy was to put as much plaster on the limb as possible. Most of my newly plastered patients needed a forklift truck to move them afterwards but their fractures were stable.

During my internship I applied for a few pathology training programmes. It seemed they weren't as enthusiastic about me as I was about them so I decided to change tack and go for my second choice, A&E. I had just moved to Dundee to take up the post when I heard from one of the pathology schemes. There had been changes in senior personnel and a letter offering me a trainee position had been delayed. I decided I might as well give A&E a go and defer making a decision until later.

Dundee Royal Infirmary was a much bigger hospital than my intern-year hospitals and therefore had all the experts who weren't available when I had worked in the peripherals. Now I found myself acting as a medical traffic warden, assessing patients and passing them on to someone who would know what to do. Much safer for the patient but a bit boring for me. The decision was made: pathology.

In 1979 I started my training. Immediately it became clear that I was more comfortable with postmortems. My first was a marathon, taking an entire day, and the hardest part was plucking up the courage to take a scalpel and cut into the body. My boss eventually lost patience: 'He's dead, you can't do any harm.' When we'd finished I still had no idea what the man had died of, until it was pointed out to me that the sticky blood I had carefully removed from blood vessels in the lungs was a pulmonary embolism, a clot that had travelled from his leg veins, to block the vessels in his lungs and cause his death. Deep vein thrombosis is a common complication of being bed bound, but since then great efforts have been made to prevent it occurring.

The hospital pathology departments in Glasgow dealt with people who had died in hospital so I was soon diagnosing heart attacks, metastasising (spreading) cancers, brain haemorrhages and blood poisoning. All natural diseases, all screwing up the body and causing death. In some cases I was surprised that someone had lived as long as they had because most of the organs were well past their best.

While I was excelling in the mortuary I was failing in the laboratory. The technicians carefully processed the pieces of tissue removed from patients to produce thin slivers stained with a variety of dyes to show the structure of the individual cells, which were floated on glass slides and presented to the pathologists on A4 size cardboard trays. So far so good. The glass slides were carefully loaded onto the microscope and the lens focused. To me, looking into the microscope was like looking into a kaleidoscope, lots of pretty colours. It was a complete mystery to me. I could not make head nor tail of what I was looking at. The only clue came on the request form accompanying the tissue because what I could see down the microscope bore no relation to what I had seen in the glass jar sent up from theatre. Another trainee who started at the same time as I did was gaily identifying not only the tissue but the pathology. This was a disaster, as far as my career prospects were concerned. Allowances are made to give trainees a chance to get the hang of things, but at some point a decision has to be made as to their suitability. I decided to adopt the policy that had worked for me during my finals: say nothing, they may think you're stupid but there is no definite proof. I was enjoying the postmortems and everyone was great: I didn't want to leave. But I was facing the possibility of my contract not being renewed at the end of six months.

And then it happened. Prepared for the usual disappointment when I put my eyes to the lenses, what I was looking at came into focus. There were uterine curettings in proliferative phase, sections of an adenocarcinoma of the bowel, perfectly normal breast tissue with no evidence of cancer and skin polyps. Game on.

The next five years were relatively uneventful and it seemed I had found my niche. The final pathology exam loomed but that was a formality and soon I was no longer a trainee. I had to start looking for a consultant histopathology position.

There was nothing on the horizon in Glasgow and I wasn't sure about my chances of getting any consultant post that came up either. While I had been a happy fit in Stobhill Hospital I knew I wasn't everyone's cup of tea. For a start I genuinely loved pathology and looked forward to work. During my training I had been sent to do a stint in the histopathology department at the Royal Infirmary in Glasgow. Those with aspirations would kill to get into the Royal or the Western. The other hospitals, including Stobhill, were regarded as inferior.

But being a doctor in a major hospital is not all roses. The only upside for me during my short time at the Royal was that none of the resident pathology trainees wanted to do the autopsies and I got to spend a lot of my time in the mortuary. That didn't dampen my spirits, which didn't go unnoticed. One Monday morning the professor of pathology looked at me and asked, 'Why are you so cheerful? It's Monday morning!' I got on to Rod, my boss back in Stobhill, and asked if I could come home. Luckily the trainee I had exchanged with was even more miserable in Stobhill than she had been at the Royal and was as desperate as I was to go back to her home department.

My other major flaw was that I didn't look like an academic. I wore stilettos and dyed my hair, with varying results. Apparently, the lab staff placed bets on what colour it would be on Monday morning. Home dyeing can be unpredictable. So I was often dismissed as rather 'flighty' even though Rod championed me. When I passed my MRCPath on the first attempt the professors had to admit, grudgingly, that I wasn't a complete airhead.

Scotland and England are not only separated by a big wall but the legal system is completely different. I wasn't aware of that. When I looked into applying for consultant positions in England I found that the autopsy system and the process of death investigation were completely different too. I vaguely remembered lectures on forensic medicine in my fourth year at university but had taken as much notice of them as I did of the lectures on tropical medicine. As I had only ever travelled as far as Majorca I wasn't sure I needed to know much about leishmaniasis.

Now I found out that in Scotland, if it was suspected that someone had died from unnatural causes, their body was spirited away to be examined by a forensic pathologist. When I asked, I was informed that there were three forensic pathologists in Glasgow. They were entirely separate from the hospital pathology departments and worked at the city mortuary in the centre of town. They dealt with road traffic deaths, hangings and overdoses, people who died in the streets and murders. In England the investigation of unnatural and sudden unexpected death was similar but the hospital pathologist carried out many of these autopsies, though suspected homicides were investigated by the forensic pathologists. By now I could do a postmortem with my eyes closed, but I had never examined anyone who had died in a fire or drowned, or has died in violent circumstances, only those who had died in hospital of natural causes. That had to be addressed if I was to have any chance of getting a consultant position in England.

I had a meeting with the professor of pathology to discuss my future. He assured me that, if I hung on, in time something might come up and there was a very good chance I would get it. Translated, that meant there was no chance unless all the trainees at the Royal and the Western hospitals were wiped out by a tsunami in the Clyde. I broached the possibility of moving south and explained that to do so successfully I needed experience of forensic pathology. He was stunned. In the mid-1980s forensic pathology had a poor reputation, to put it mildly: forensic pathologists were regarded as failed histopathologists, dealing with the deaths of the dregs of society. He recovered sufficiently to say that he would see what could be done and I was dismissed. My immediate thought was that I'd done it now. I'd gone from being a frivolous pathologist to toxic. Later that day he phoned to say I could join the forensic department for two weeks. I was delighted. But he hadn't finished: he followed up with a potential job offer. Would I be interested in a career in forensic pathology? There was a vacant position they couldn't fill. This time I was the one stunned to silence. I thanked him for the generous offer but said that two weeks was fine. Little did I know that that phone call had sealed my fate.

A couple of weeks later I set off for the city mortuary. I knew I could perform an autopsy better than most of the trainees but I wasn't sure if I could deal with the mangled messes I would encounter. I had vivid enough memories of A&E:

people screaming in pain, injuries that the surgeons had no idea how to fix, and those were the lucky ones with a fighting chance of survival.

The living have to travel to be treated, while the dead were taken to a building five minutes from the main shopping street in Glasgow. I always said that the only perk in my job was free parking in the centre of Glasgow during the Christmas period. From the outside the mortuary resembled a public toilet, an austere building. Inside it was all off-white tiles and functional. Easy clean. However, the welcome was friendly – the three mortuary attendants were obviously delighted to have a new face, a female face. I was offered tea and cake. I thought that this must have been a special concession for my visit but found that this was the norm and I became very fond of my 'wee cup of tea', especially when things got a bit fraught. Jackie, Fenton and Alec would become my mortuary uncles, looking out for me for the next few years.

My immediate impression was of how quiet the place was. There was also the very pungent stench of carbolic soap, Jackie's favourite cleaning product. The public areas were dimly lit, I thought to create an ambience of calm for grieving relatives, but I soon discovered that another of Jackie's quirks was a frugal approach to the running of the mortuary, which included removal of alternate light bulbs to save electricity. I'm sure the fathers of Glasgow City Council would have been delighted to know that one employee was looking after their interests. That would become a constant battle, Fenton being my main ally, fitting light bulbs and emptying vast quantities of liquid carbolic soap down the drains. Which was probably a good thing when I think of all the other stuff that was flushed down.

Professor Watson was head of the forensic department, a dapper gentleman, always attired in a pinstripe suit, even when called out in the small hours of the night. He had silver hair, wore rimless glasses and had an English accent. Just the type of authoritative figure the courts love. I remembered him from the lectures he had given when I was a student. He explained how the system worked but I just wanted to get into the dissection room. I had no idea how I was going to react. I hoped I wouldn't end up on the floor, as I had at my first encounters with patients and their blood.

Well, first, this was a million miles away from the hospital mortuaries, which largely emulated operating theatres, all shiny stainless steel, with state-of-the-art ventilation systems purifying the air, changing areas with showers, all mod cons. This mortuary had a rather Dickensian charm. There was a single makeshift 'changing' room used by all, which in reality was the storeroom and passage into the postmortem room. Instead of theatre scrubs to change into, disposable aprons and gloves, I was shown a pile of slightly tatty green linen gowns, reusable wipe-'clean' plastic aprons and an assortment of gloves, all in a large size. Thirty-odd years later I still find that mortuaries are designed for tall people with large hands and feet. The professor had his own wipe-clean apron, with 'PROF' written across the top in indelible felt-tip marker. I had to make do with one marked 'CAD'. Much later I was to learn that CAD stood for Coronary Artery Disease, the favoured diagnosis of a pathologist who assisted on occasions. Of course the apron was far too long and required a bit of Heath Robinson ingenuity so I didn't trip over it and knock myself out on the marble floor.

Suitably attired, we walked straight from there into the postmortem room. It was big and bright with three large white porcelain tables, each designed to take two bodies, which wouldn't be condoned now, and shouldn't have been then, but, as I was to discover over the course of my career, there was no money for the dead. It was only as forensic science became such a vital tool in criminal investigations that the city mortuary had to be upgraded due to the risk of contamination of DNA evidence.

There were four bodies, in varying stages of dissection, waiting for our attention, each with its own pitiful story, and all waiting for us to explore and discover what had caused their death. There was a fire death, two elderly 'drop-deads', and a relatively young person, the first of the drug addicts I would meet. Like Alice, I had fallen down a rabbit hole and discovered a world previously unknown to me. Like Alice, I would meet interesting, odd and wonderful people, alive and dead: a world I never wanted to leave.

For the next thirteen years I honed my craft in Glasgow. I carried out over five thousand postmortems, mostly sudden, accidental or suicidal deaths, but this was Glasgow so there were a fair number of murders. They were mainly stabbings, with anything from one to more than a hundred stab wounds. The implements ranged from the innocent pencil to the ornamental samurai sword, a common feature on living-room walls in 1980s Glasgow. The next most common method was blunt trauma, principally head injuries due to punching, kicking or being struck with a large weighty object, such as a hammer, a wheel brace or a rock – anything at hand, really.

A few years later guns entered the fray. The Glasgow gangsters now had a new weapon at their disposal and the forensic pathologists had to up their game too. I visited the forensic department in Belfast to get up to speed with shootings, which were commonplace during the 'Troubles' in Northern Ireland. In addition to these methods there was a smattering of strangulations.

In between we lectured to medical and law students and set up a training programme for anyone involved in the forensics industry, from nurses and doctors to firefighters and barristers.

Forensic pathology is all-consuming. You can't do it half-heartedly: long hours, lost weekends and missed celebrations are the norm. Your colleagues become your friends, your family has to be understanding, your partner becomes a part-time single parent and you eat, sleep and breathe death.

In 1998 I left Glasgow for Ireland to join Professor Jack Harbison in Dublin as deputy state pathologist. It was the same job I had been doing but suddenly I was thrown into the public arena in a way that was seen as unseemly in the UK. In Scotland the forensic pathologists were known within the small circle of those involved in death investigation and the general public had little or no interest in who we were or even what we did.

I had known Jack for many years and he had often regaled us with tales of his time as state pathologist. On one occasion he had visited Glasgow as external examiner for the forensic medicine examination for medical students. He got his flight times wrong and a car sent to pick him up came back empty. Later, when he arrived at Glasgow airport, there was no welcoming party, so, naturally, he went up to a policeman and asked him to take him to Professor Vanesis's office. The policeman had no idea who Jack or Vanesis were, but agreed to contact his senior officer. Eventually they worked out that Jack was trying to find the forensic medicine department and so they called us. Jack arrived full of bonhomie, amazed that no one in Glasgow, a slight exaggeration, knew who the professor of forensic medicine was. 'Sure, everyone in Ireland knows me.' Of course they do, Jack!

Fast forward a few years. Post the high-profile Sophie Toscan du Plantier murder in west Cork, 1996, the realisation came that one forensic pathologist could not be expected to investigate every suspicious death in the entire country: Jack contacted me to see if I would be interested in joining him in Ireland. I said I would think about it and offered to pop over to get an idea of the situation. I arrived at Dublin airport, no sign of Jack. Tit for tat! A call came over the Tannoy: 'Will Dr Cassidy come to the information desk.' Expecting to hear Jack was running late, I was surprised to find two gardaí who told me Professor Harbison was at a scene and had requested that I be brought there.

I was bundled into the back of the garda car and we sped off through Dublin to Grangegorman, where two women lay dead. Before I knew it I was having conversations with the forensic scientists about bloody fingerprints: which was more important – DNA analysis or identifying the fingerprint? That was an ongoing discussion in Glasgow too. This was a horrendous double murder and little did I realise that it would not be solved for many years. My visit sealed the deal: Ireland it was to be. It also confirmed that everyone knew who Jack was.

So, the second phase of my career was in Ireland in the Office of the State Pathologist. Same job but different in many ways.

The Irish are obsessed with death. Attending funerals is a national sport, while in Scotland one has to have a legitimate link to the deceased: only family and close friends get to partake in the steak pie breakfast, the highlight of the event. In Ireland there are death notices announced on local radio and, rather than check your horoscope or do the crossword, people check the paper to see if anyone within a ten-mile radius has died, as that seems to be a legitimate enough reason to attend a funeral, others being, 'I knew his cousin', or 'My granny lived round the corner'. I remember when my own mother died we knew everyone in the church apart from one person, a representative from the Department of Justice. Nice thought but totally unnecessary at a Scottish funeral. He didn't stay for the steak pie. But thank you, Noel.

This fascination with death translates into

press coverage of deaths, not just murders, which was why Jack was such a public figure. While he relished his 'fame', I have always felt uneasy at the intrusion. Try shopping in the local supermarket, which I know Jack never did, and people coming over to chat, which is lovely, but I know they're checking out the contents of my trolley. It's almost enough to make you teetotal. But not quite.

For the next twenty years I devoted my time and energy to investigating suspicious deaths in Ireland. During this time forensic science progressed and the role of the pathologist changed. The attendance of the forensic pathologist at the scene of a death became largely redundant from the investigators' point of view, but I never refused to go. Advances in trauma care, and an upgraded road system which led to an improvement in paramedics' response times, meant the severely injured were rapidly transported to hospital and resuscitated successfully, and the 'simple' cases – the single stab wound and some head injuries – never got to us, and so the cases we dealt with became more complex. Despite that, the process has remained the same over the years and, while mortuaries have been upgraded, the pathologist still relies on a sharp knife, a pair of scissors and a saw, electric preferred.

It wasn't always thus. The rapid changes in the forensic investigation of deaths in my lifetime mirror the advances in science and technology which affect all our lives. But, as with all aspects of modern living, the reality is that the evolution of the process of investigation of deaths took centuries.

2

A Lesson in Death

AS THE PROCESS OF INVESTIGATION of deaths evolved, the role of the forensic pathologist emerged and we entered a new era of understanding how death comes about.

Until fairly recently, examination of the body as part of an investigation of the cause and circumstances of a death was more out of curiosity than an intent to uncover crime. The first recorded postmortem of a victim of homicide was Julius Caesar. Twenty-three stab wounds were described and the fatal wound was to his chest, piercing the aorta: '*Et tu Brute.*' Pretty definitive result, even by today's standards. However, in general, up until the 1100s death was literally just the end of life. Move on.

For eight hundred years, after the Normans landed in Ireland in the late 1100s, Ireland lived in the shadow of English rule so the law of England was adopted in Ireland. Even post-independence Ireland clung to some relics of the past, including the coronial system for investigating deaths.

If there was little desire to look after the interests of the individual, particularly the poor, in England, the Irish were likely to suffer even worse treatment. Citizens expected their rulers to look after them, defend their interests. But, of course, that came at a cost. The Crown in England realised that investigating the deaths of citizens at home and across the water could be advantageous: while ostensibly looking after people's interests, in reality they exploited the situation, seizing the assets of the deceased, possibly the forerunner of inheritance tax, and fining the perpetrators of crime. The person appointed to carry out the royal orders was the coroner. A cross between the Sheriff of Nottingham and Friar Tuck, he pocketed the assets of a beloved husband while proffering condolences to the bereaved wife.

In 1194, the Articles of Eyre cemented the position of the coroner's role in death investigation in England, and therefore, by default, also in

Ireland. In England the coroner had to confirm the identification of the deceased and determine the cause and manner of death, which they did by holding an inquest. In those days, and until fairly recent times, the conduct of an inquest could not have been more different from the sanitised court hearing of today.

The then coroner and his jury, a hotchpotch of local worthies, gathered in a public place, and had a look at the body, the equivalent of the modern postmortem examination. The local public house was often the only building with a surface large enough to hold a body for examination, as well as accommodate the jury. In those early days, neither the coroner nor his jury had any medical training, but a consensus opinion as to the likely cause of death was reached: simple enough if the unfortunate had been trampled by a horse or beaten to death in a drunken fury. Job done.

Strangely, or maybe not, this practice opened up opportunities in Ireland and the role of the publican became entwined with that of the undertaker. And this was made official in 1846 by the Coroner's Act. In Ireland during the Famine the number of deaths overwhelmed the existing medical services and facilities: today this would be classified as a Major Disaster. To cope with the situation the Coroner's Act decreed that dead bodies were to be brought to the nearest public house where they would be stored in the beer cellars, the only cold-storage facilities available, until an inquest could be held. The 1962 Coroner's Act superseded this, but by then funeral homes were springing up, a more decorous resting place for the deceased, although many publicans retained their interest in this side of their business. In rural Ireland today there are still publicans-cum-undertakers-cum-local shopkeepers. Although now the bodies are no longer stored in the beer cellars, the publican can offer a full service, from funeral arrangements to the wake. An Irish solution to an Irish problem, and it's legal. Spar just couldn't compete.

In addition, the historic coroner had the authority to collect death duties and to confiscate the property of a felon on behalf of the Crown. The reality was that identifying the deceased and establishing the cause of death was just a means to an end: getting their hands on the money.

Of course, if the death was natural or accidental, and no one could be held responsible, there was little money in it for the coroner or his master. In general, people had precious little in the way of assets, and as coroners weren't paid but relied on getting a cut of the proceeds, it is not surprising that the system became corrupt. Over time the emphasis of inquiries changed, and by 1500, the sole function of the coroner was to hold inquests into violent deaths. Well, that was where the money was. The introduction of a fee for the holding of an inquest was an attempt to ensure that the coroners were honest and moral in their investigation of deaths. The coroner as we know him or her today was born.

Scotland has long striven for independence from England. It has spurned the English legal system, even though it is part of the United Kingdom. Lawyers trained in Scotland cannot set up shop in England, and vice versa. Therefore, Scotland developed its own system of death investigation derived from Europe. There is no coroner in Scotland: the person responsible for investigating death is the procurator fiscal. Although the role is similar to that of the coroner, the main distinction is that the procurator fiscal also acts as the public prosecutor. This official's role is first mentioned in the 1400s, long after establishment of the coroner. In those early days, the procurator fiscal had a duty to seek out and prosecute 'delinquents and disobedient people'. They were 'policing' the population, the forerunners of today's police, and when the Glasgow constabulary were established in 1800, they had to comply with the direction of the procurator fiscal. This position was ratified in the Sheriff Courts (Scotland) Act of 1867 by which the procurator fiscal was given full responsibility for the prosecution of all criminal acts in Scotland.

By the 1830s, in England and Ireland, the coroner had the power to instruct a doctor to examine the deceased. Similar advances in death investigation were being made in Scotland. The medical postmortem examination, or autopsy, was instituted as part of the investigation, which introduced a new member to the investigating team, the pathologist.

In Europe, since the 1200s, medical schools had been granted access to the bodies of criminals for anatomy demonstrations. These were performed in operating theatres, the medical students forming the audience. Famously, Leonardo da Vinci and Michelangelo performed such autopsies: anatomy was of more interest to the artists than to the medics. Picasso would never have had a career as a plastic surgeon. Over the next few hundred years, as more and more bodies were dissected and disease patterns were recognised, based on the appearance of the internal organs, doctors' understanding of the human body, how it is affected by illness and disease, and how illness and disease cause death, grew apace, heralding the beginning of modern medicine. The anatomists were the precursors of the pathologist.

Anatomists such as John Hunter, who established an anatomy school in London in the 1760s, catalogued their findings by retaining the abnormal organs, which were preserved in glass specimen containers – a museum of human innards. They also kept 'curiosities', such as conjoined twins and foetuses with fatal congenital abnormalities. A visit to the anatomy museum was a must for a medical student.

However, medical schools struggled to acquire bodies for teaching their students, which led to some unscrupulous practices. In 1827, in Edinburgh, the enterprising William Burke and William Hare saw an opportunity to further science, and make a few pounds. They supplied bodies to Dr Robert Knox, professor of pathology at the Edinburgh Medical School. When legitimate bodies, those of hanged criminals, the deceased with no family, or the poor who couldn't afford to dispose of their dead, weren't available they disinterred fresh corpses. This was not without risk, and was hard work, so eventually they took things into their own hands: they suffocated, smothered or strangled the vulnerable and incapacitated, or drunk. All in all, they were said to have dispatched sixteen people before their career ended in 1828. There may be honour among thieves but obviously not among murderers: Hare gave evidence against Burke, who was hanged and his body duly delivered to the anatomy department for dissection. A perfect ending and perhaps his only altruistic act, albeit posthumous.

When the truth became known of Burke and Hare's activities, a public outcry followed, which led to an attempt to regulate the 'industry' with the 1832 Anatomy Act. Medical schools were now officially licensed to dissect donated bodies. However, there are always loopholes and, while this protected the rich, the poor were still vulnerable to exploitation: selling your granny to the anatomy department was still worth a few quid to the grieving relatives.

The major breakthrough in the investigation

of death and disease was the introduction of the microscope in the 1830s. Now anatomists and medics were able to delve even deeper into the body. Not only could they look at whole organs, they could see that each was a collection of smaller units forming distinctive patterns and shapes. This was the beginning of histopathology, of determining the cause of death and understanding illness and disease.

In 1832 an Asiatic cholera epidemic rampaged across continents causing death and destruction. It led to more than three thousand deaths in Glasgow alone. In order to determine the global effect of this disease, public health officials recognised that postmortem examinations on all deaths occurring during this time could help them identify deaths due to the infection rather than from some other cause, which in turn would help them determine the exact numbers affected, how the disease spread and why some people were more vulnerable to it than others.

The success of this instigated a push for postmortems in the investigation of all deaths. But who was going to perform them? Well, pathologists with an interest in public health, of course. Unfortunately, they did not exist.

A new department was set up in universities in Scotland and London: the Department of Medical Jurisprudence and Public Health. It was a hybrid, law and medicine colliding in the public interest. Could hybrid doctors be found? The first incumbents of the professorial posts usually had an interest in either medical jurisprudence or public health, not both, and even then, some preferred teaching students to providing an autopsy service or engaging in research. The unholy alliance between the two disparate disciplines limped on for some considerable time with varying degrees of success. But a split was inevitable.

In the 1900s forensic medicine suddenly took centre stage. This was probably fuelled by the public's interest in the fictional Sherlock Holmes. Forensic pathologists moved into the public arena and became the celebrities of the day: the new medical detectives, who included Bernard Spilsbury in London, the Glaisters in Glasgow, the Littlejohns and Sydney Smith in Edinburgh. This was the era of the medical showman. Their cases became legendary, as did their gladiatorial sparring in court, one against another. The public galleries in courts were full to overflowing. By far the best way to be part of the spectacle was to be in the midst of it.

When they weren't preening themselves in front of the court or the press, those eminent pathologists were laying the foundations of forensic death investigation as we now know it. They were fledgling investigators, without the benefit of the experts I surround myself with today. The forensic pathologist was a Jack-of-all-trades: pathologist, scientist, toxicologist and psychiatrist.

John Glaister senior set the stage for the Glasgow Department of Forensic Medicine and Toxicology that was my home for many years. He produced a textbook, *Medical Jurisprudence*, in 1902, which was innovative as it used photographs to illustrate the text. It was updated fairly regularly, particularly as forensic science progressed. His son, John Glaister junior, had a keen interest in forensic science, and was instrumental in introducing the new tests on blood, hair and fibres routinely used in cases today. It would be another twenty years in Glasgow before the service fragmented, when pathologists, police and scientists would diverge and specialise, and forensic pathologists would have to admit that they were not experts in all matters forensic.

Those professors of forensic medicine became household names mainly because of the high-profile cases they were involved with. Bernard Spilsbury gave evidence in the 'Brides in the Bath' case. A serial husband disposed of his wives by drowning them in the bath. If all of your wives drown in that manner it's more than a little suspicious: Spilsbury was not convinced that the deaths were coincidental and accidental, and demonstrated how the victims were grasped by the ankle and pulled under the water. The coincidence theory may have been hard to accept, but the physical evidence to support the new one was a bit flimsy too. It was really no more than a theory, but delivered to his audience, the jury, with such aplomb. He was probably right but today the court requires more than theatrics to convict someone of murder.

His successor, Keith Simpson, was involved in the 'Acid Bath Murder'. A man committed a series of murders of middle-aged women. He successfully disposed of the bodies in acid but his last victim was his undoing. He dissolved the body as best he could in a tub of sulphuric acid in the basement of her house, but as there was no drainage he scooped up the sludge and deposited it on a pile of rubble in the backyard. During the course of an inquiry into the woman's disappearance, part of a foot was found in the rubble. Spilsbury identified, in addition, twenty-eight pounds of human fat, gallstones and part of a denture, later identified by the woman's dentist, sufficient, before DNA analysis became available, to identify her.

While those early days of forensic pathology were exciting, the lack of scientific research meant that sometimes the forensic pathologists made rather sweeping statements that went unchallenged and likely strengthened the police case, securing a conviction and the judicial death of the alleged perpetrator. Now such arrogance would not be allowed to go unchecked.

As forensic science blossomed, the self-assured forensic pathologist, who convinced public and jury of the accused's guilt, even if it wasn't an open and shut case, was no longer needed. Now the police would have physical evidence that could link the accused with the deceased. Now the emphasis was on forensic science, not the forensic pathologist. Now forensic pathology had to get serious.

3

Death Scene

DR HAROLD SHIPMAN FAMOUSLY DISPATCHED a couple of hundred patients, injections of morphine being his choice of murder weapon. As the deceased person's general practitioner, and likely the doctor called in to confirm death, he had the power to thwart and control any investigations into these deaths.

If a doctor is of the opinion that a death is due to natural causes, there is no need for further investigation, particularly when death occurs at home, or, as in some of Shipman's cases, in the doctor's surgery. Thus, by certifying these deaths as due to natural causes, Dr Shipman ensured there would be no further enquiries.

Morphine overdose was not listed as the principal cause of death on the medical certificate, a legal document issued by doctors when a death is due to natural causes. Who would question a doctor? Why would he lie? And who is going to say something to the contrary? Are the family going to ask for a second opinion?

Once a doctor issues this certificate, families can register the death and make their arrangements. If it had not been for a vigilant undertaker questioning the death rate at Shipman's practice his actions would have remained undetected. The integrity of any investigation is dependent on the integrity of each link in the chain. Dr Shipman was the weak link in the death-investigation chain, and he ensured he was the last link so his actions were not subject to scrutiny. The reliance on human honesty was always the main flaw in the investigation of deaths.

In England that weakness has been addressed by introducing a medical examiner system to investigate all deaths: now there should be nowhere for doctors to hide. Every death will be scrutinised by an independent doctor, whether at home, in hospital or in a care home, no matter the circumstances. If there are any queries regarding a death, the treatment of a patient by medical staff – in or out of hospital – or any family concerns, they will be thoroughly investigated.

In Ireland, in contrast to the UK, the coroners have always been conscious of the fallibility of the system, hence there has always been a higher postmortem rate. Thankfully in Ireland this does not impede families' arrangements for funerals; most bodies are released within a couple of days. In the UK in the event of a postmortem families typically have to wait a couple of weeks to have a body returned. The key is finding a system that works, safeguarding the population.

The process of death investigation has evolved over the years. Every country has similar procedures. Only the personnel in charge differ: it might be the police, the judiciary or a coroner (or equivalent). The system is designed to prevent homicides, in particular, going undetected. But its robustness depends on the honesty and diligence of each person involved in investigating the death, and includes family, friends, doctors and other medical personnel, as well as the police and other investigators, making any concerns known to the relevant authorities.

The examination of the deceased at the scene

of death is the first chance to get things right or wrong. Dr Shipman attended the death scenes of his patients. It was in his interest to prevent further enquiries and he successfully ensured that the investigations ground to a halt at the scene, assuring the authorities that there was no need for any further action. In most instances those called to attend the scene of a death make the right decision. Mercifully, there are few Dr Shipmans.

The first decision to be made is whether or not this is a straightforward death due to natural causes or if it requires further investigation. In natural deaths, burial or cremation will follow rapidly, particularly in Ireland. If there is any uncertainty as to the actual cause of death, or the circumstances of the death, a more in-depth enquiry will be made, which may lead to a postmortem examination being carried out; phase two of the process. If something was overlooked at the scene, this is where it should be rectified.

Surely an external and internal examination of the entire body will identify anything unusual and, most importantly, the cause of death? One would hope so, but it depends on the thoroughness of the examination and the expertise of the doctor carrying out the postmortem. So, it's not fool-proof.

I cannot comment on how many homicides remain undetected following a postmortem, only on the diligence of those pathologists who brought some deaths to my attention due to an unexpected finding or findings that didn't quite fit the information they had been given. Many of these deaths were resolved satisfactorily but a few were indeed murders, proving that the system works, most of the time.

One such incident involved a family. On Christmas morning in 2008 I was busy getting breakfast ready. Santa had been and my grown children, 19 and 20 years old, were happily squabbling over the number of selection boxes each had. I was on call so had my ear to the radio, as ever waiting for breaking news of death and destruction, death never taking a holiday.

I heard that there had been a house fire in the Kilkenny area and a mother and her two children had died. Shortly after, I had a call from the gardaí dealing with the situation. They informed me they weren't treating the deaths of the Whelan family as 'suspicious': probably the Christmas tree lights had been left on, causing an accidental fire; a very sad accident, it was supposed. I got on with my day, always on the alert, waiting for a call out but relaxed enough to enjoy Christmas dinner. Christmas Day is the best day of the year, in my mind.

The next morning an apologetic garda called me. There had been a worrying development since he had last spoken to me. The local pathologist had come in early to carry out postmortems on the family, mindful of the time of year and how important it would be for relatives to have the bodies back and start the grieving process. The pathologist had completed the examinations of the children first and found black smoke lining their airways: death due to the suffocating effect of smoke and the toxic gases from the fire.

However, the mother showed no blackening of the airways. The pathologist was concerned, and informed the gardaí that this was an unusual finding: she might have died before the fire took hold. Could I look at Mrs Whelan? Of course, I said, but I would examine all three bodies and required the assistance of a full forensic team.

That afternoon, I was in the mortuary at Waterford Regional Hospital, still hoping for a reasonable explanation, that this had been, as everyone had thought, a tragic accident. Perhaps she had had a heart attack and collapsed before, or at the sight of, a fire in her home. Perhaps she had been drinking or had taken drugs. The postmortem would show signs of these.

I was largely left to my own devices as I set about my business. Most of the dissection of Mrs Whelan had already been carried out. Sure enough, the trachea was free from sticky black soot. But within a few minutes of starting my examination I found an injury to her throat: her Adam's apple was damaged. There was bruising of the muscles of the neck, which couldn't be explained by the aborted examination and, most worrying of all, her thyroid cartilage and hyoid bone were fractured. There was no doubt in my mind that she had been strangled. The room stilled as I asked the investigating gardaí to come over to the table.

Their cheery tales of Christmas Day stopped mid-sentence when I stated that all was not well. That Mrs Whelan had not died in a fire: she was already dead when the fire started. She had been murdered. The enormity of the situation dawned on everyone present. If Mrs Whelan had been murdered, the fire could have been started deliberately to conceal her death, and therefore, as her children had died from the fire fumes, all three deaths were murders.

Luckily the scene had not been disturbed any more than had been required to remove all three bodies. I had no doubt about the cause of the mother's death, and agreed with the pathologist that the fire had caused the children's deaths, but only a full forensic examination of the scene would confirm that the fire had been started deliberately. The forensic team returned to the scene.

I continued my examination of Mrs Whelan. Having found internal evidence of strangulation, I began to look for other signs. Was she throttled, hands squeezing her neck, or was a ligature pulled tight around it? Also, strangulation is not usually premeditated but tends to happen in certain situations. More women than men are strangled and in the majority of cases this is linked to sexual activity. I looked for evidence of recent sexual intercourse: this helps to establish the circumstances leading to the final act, but there may also be forensic evidence to identify the perpetrator. Locard's Principle: every contact leaves a trace. There was clear evidence of recent sexual activity. In general, a doctor cannot determine whether or not sexual activity is consensual, unless there are savage injuries. But it was clear from subsequent events that Sharon Whelan was not a willing partner.

Back at the scene it became obvious to the Technical Bureau that the fire had been deliberately started. They were shown the position of the bodies when found; Sharon Whelan had been face down on the floor of the bedroom, one child had been in a cot and the other on a bed. The findings suggested that Sharon had likely been killed in the living room and moved into the bedroom. The postmortems on the children had shown no evidence of injuries and they appeared to have died from the fire fumes. The neighbours, who had noticed smoke coming from the house, must have been distraught that, although they could see the children inside, they couldn't save them. The window was smashed in the attempts to get access but by that time it was too late: it doesn't take long for fire fumes to snuff out a little life. No one could have done anything to prevent the children dying other than the man who eventually admitted starting the fire after he had strangled their mother. He said he was worried that she would let their 'relationship' be known.

*

Every death investigation starts with a phone call. Depending on the hour of the day, or night, the police/gardaí, procurator fiscal/coroner, or my office might call me. 'The scene' is where a criminal incident may have taken place and, in the case of a potential murder, where a body is found. This is where a murder investigation starts. An incident may have been witnessed – commonly a drunken brawl in the pub or on the street; someone comes home to find the body of a family member or friend; a dog-walker comes across a body; or the police are given information which leads to the discovery of the body of someone reported missing. There are as many scenarios of discovery as there are bodies.

Once a body is discovered, a call is made to the police, which sets a chain of events in motion. Depending on the content of the call – an obvious violent death, such as a shooting incident, for example – a full forensic murder investigation may be mobilised immediately. In other instances of sudden or unexpected death, which are less obviously murder, an advance party of local police will attend to assess the situation. It will be for them to decide whether or not the death can be treated as unexplained – requiring a postmortem examination, and possibly the forensic examination of the scene depending on the outcome – or a potential murder, in which case the full forensic team will be required from the outset.

Once it is decided that the death is 'suspicious', all relevant parties will be notified and expected to attend: detectives, forensic scientists, finger-printers, photographers and the forensic pathologist. Any potential scene is locked down, out comes the police tape, entry by invitation only.

In Ireland, the gardaí must inform the coroner, the representative of the state who is legally responsible for the investigation of the death, that a body has been discovered that requires full forensic investigation: the coroner has the power to instruct any of the state agencies to assist in the investigation of a death. But the coroner's role is limited to determining the identity of the victim and their personal details, as well as where, when and how they died. Importantly, they cannot apportion blame for a death – in other words, they can't identify any person or persons responsible for the death and certainly can't prosecute them. So, while in the initial stages of the investigation all of the key players are working at the behest of the coroner, what happens next hinges on the 'how': how did the person die? Breath is held until the pathologist's final cut. This is the only moment in any death investigation in which the pathologist takes centre stage: is it murder or not?

If it is not murder, the coroner retains control and may hold an inquest. If it is murder, the police will continue the investigation, but the coroner now takes a back seat. Once all the forensic investigations have been completed, and the police have a suspect in mind, they will present the evidence to the office of the Director of Public Prosecutions, the DPP, responsible for prosecuting criminal offenders, including murderers. It is the DPP's decision whether or not there is sufficient evidence for a case to be pursued through the courts, with a view to convicting someone for the crime.

Back at the beginning, after the discovery of the body, all state agencies deemed necessary will congregate at the scene of the death. The police, the forensic investigators and the pathologists all view the scene from a different perspective: the police are gathering information regarding the incident leading to the death, the forensic investigators are looking for physical evidence linking the deceased and possible assailants, and the pathologist is mainly concerned with the body and how they died.

In reality there may be more than one scene of relevance in any murder investigation: where a body is found, the place someone was last seen alive, where an assault took place, where an injured party moved to, or was moved to, prior to their collapse, any vehicle involved in the transportation of the perpetrators or the victim. It is much easier if an assault followed by death is confined to one place and the perpetrator is caught red-handed. Otherwise the forensic team, in particular, have to spread themselves thin. As far as the pathologist is concerned, the body is the scene.

The first police officer responding to the call has the important duty to secure the scene and protect all vital forensic evidence. They must keep everyone out other than the relevant personnel. No one wants the scene contaminated. In the first instance that means taping off the area. In Scotland it means closing off a road and as large an area as possible. In Ireland it means stopping people coming up the garden path: at times the press get too close for comfort. Before I became familiar with garda photographers in Ireland I arrived at one scene and was told to wait outside until the team were ready. To pass the time I chatted with a photographer beside me, only a few feet from the body. When I was waved over, I motioned to the photographer to follow and was shocked when he told me that he was press, not police. Thankfully, we had talked about everything but the death.

There is nothing more frustrating than arriving at a scene to be told the body is in an ambulance on the way to the mortuary. For me the most pressing issue is that there are many police, and even several forensic teams, but there is only one pathologist on call at weekends when there may be more than one death treated as suspicious. And they may be at either end of the country. That was why I sometimes got a little tetchy if I was left waiting for the forensic team to arrive or if they took for ever before I could go in to a scene. I was worried that if something happened elsewhere in the country people would be hanging around waiting for me. I hate wasting people's time. Time isn't money for me, but it can potentially cause unnecessary delays in deciding what direction an investigation will take: murder or not.

Until I see the body, I have no idea what is relevant at the scene of the death: bloodstains, potential weapons or any disturbance. I've been fooled.

In one instance I had a look at a body lying on the living-room floor of a tenement flat in Glasgow. The victim had been stabbed when a fight broke out during a drinking session. There was a single stab wound on his chest, which appeared as though it had been caused by a broad blade. In an effort to help identify the possible weapon, I had a look around the flat.

The body was lying in front of the sofa, which had seen better days, brown Dralon, ripped and stained, and spotted with cigarette burns. The coffee table was covered with glasses and beer cans, and ashtrays overflowed with cigarette butts. The curtains were drawn and the room was illuminated by a bare bulb dangling from the ceiling. The carpet, colour long since concealed by food, drink and ash ground into the pile, showed only a small pool of blood oozing out from under the body, but there was no sign of a knife around the body. In the kitchen bin bags were bursting with beer cans and vodka bottles, and which also covered all the surfaces. On the table there was a loaf and a tub of margarine. A few knives lay in the sink but none showed any bloodstaining and most were crusted with food.

The bedroom was furnished only with a stained mattress and a chair, which functioned as part wardrobe, part laundry basket. There was no blood and nothing much else of interest. Which left the bathroom. I am usually reluctant to enter bathrooms in these circumstances. They are rarely pleasant. In this case the bath panel had been kicked in and was lying half under the bath. The porcelain sink was smashed and there was blood on the walls and the curtain at the window. The toilet seat had been wrenched from its hinges and the flush handle was on the floor. The pan was full to brimming. This appeared to have been the scene of a fight and possibly where the fight broke out.

Could the blood in the bathroom be from the deceased and, if so, could he have managed to get from the bathroom to the living room after he had been stabbed? There was no evidence of a trail but small drops of blood could easily have been concealed by the detritus on the carpets. I hoped the postmortem might answer this question.

When the flat owner had sobered up enough to be questioned by the police, his recollection of the events leading to his best pal being fatally stabbed by his other best pal were rather hazy. With friends like these . . . ! He was quite sure that whatever had happened had taken place in the living room: the bathroom had been trashed a couple of weeks earlier. The blood there belonged to another of his drinking buddies. A red herring of sorts. The knife was never recovered, another unwanted addition to the River Clyde along with the innumerable shopping trolleys.

My role at the scene is to examine the body where it lies. I'm looking for any marks or injuries that might be relevant to the death: the head injury due to a blow from a hammer rather than the head injury caused when the deceased collapsed onto the ground or floor. Within a few minutes of entering a potential crime scene I can usually assess whether or not murder is likely. Of course, that comes from experience. I have visited hundreds of scenes, inside, outside, in and on the banks of rivers, washed up from the seas, up hills and down dales.

Some terrain is easier to navigate than others. Although indoor scenes are dry and relatively warm, the living conditions of some people are startling and, in some cases, heartbreaking. It's a rare occurrence for a call to the posh side of town.

The rich are not immune to death and destruction, but violence seems to occur less often in those circles. You wouldn't believe the number of people who live in less than ideal circumstances mainly due to lack of money. Some are not equipped physically or mentally to cope and don't know how to look after themselves and their family. Poverty and squalor are a way of life and it's very difficult to haul yourself out of it. What effect must that have on your sense of self-worth? Perhaps if the jury visited the home where the crime took place they might have a bit more compassion for the accused.

While there are challenges reaching bodies in tricky situations outdoors, that is preferable to the claustrophobic atmosphere indoors which has the effect of amplifying the sights and smells, not just of death, but the stench of living: the kitchen piled with dirty plates and pans, food rotting where it was left, bathrooms used for anything other than the intended purpose. The smell of death, while it makes the others at the scene gag, to me is perfectly normal, not pleasant but understandable. It's science, not a blatant disregard for cleanliness. But even I will admit that recent death is better than months of decay.

Thankfully, full protective clothing is now mandatory when entering a potential crime scene. In my early days you kept your hands in your pockets and tried not to brush against anything. You had to tiptoe around blood, vomit and faeces, animal and human, on the floor. Luckily, as I was usually smaller than anyone else, one of my colleagues could grab hold of me and keep me upright if I slid. I learned early that there was no point in wearing anything that couldn't be thrown into the washing machine or the bin, think Primark not Prada. Only after DNA analysis became mainstream did full protective clothing become *de rigueur*, but not to protect me, but to protect the forensic evidence.

All of the protective clothing donned at the scene is supplied by the Technical Bureau, the team of guards specifically trained to attend crime scenes to document, collect and preserve evidence. They include experts in photography, fingerprints and ballistics. Years ago this was largely a male domain but more and more female guards have joined. Still, though, whoever orders the protective clothing, being frugal, as is appropriate when it comes to public funds, requests sizes that will fit the majority, XL and XXL. Occasionally a size

L will slip through the net and I am offered it, nay, presented with it, as is befitting of such a rare commodity. At a scene, I'm the little one with the crotch of the white suit around the shins, looking like a deflated Michelin man.

No matter my opinion on the circumstances of a death, based on my assessment of the scene, there will always be a full postmortem and all forensic tests will be carried out. The sooner the police know what they are dealing with, the sooner the investigation can be moved forward. A warm body means a warm trail, more likely to have a successful outcome. I admit that I must be very annoying at the scene: I want to get to the body; I want to see what the issues are. I get frustrated by the processes that are crucial to the investigation but which seem to take for ever.

Sometimes safety is the deciding factor as to when we get access to the scene, particularly with fire deaths, but, unlike Northern Ireland, there is no threat of incendiary devices or booby traps. Having to check under my car each morning might make me reconsider my career.

In Glasgow the police would expect the pathologist to attend a scene within an hour of a body being discovered. They took great pride in the death being 'wrapped up' before the press got wind of it, even if it meant traipsing out in the middle of the night, which was common there, most violent crimes happening after the pubs shut. Late opening is a real pain for forensic pathologists.

In the 1980s, before mobile phones, we had pagers. This was fine if you were near a landline, but invariably the pager would buzz when I was in the car travelling from one mortuary to another. It was then a scramble to find a phone box and contact the police or the office. The introduction of the mobile phone revolutionised our working life, but not necessarily in a good way. This made contacting the pathologist easier but it meant lugging around something the size, and weight, of a brick. More importantly, we were now instantly available 24/7.

About this time, I developed a telephone phobia. To this day, every time a phone rings I am on high alert. I am often terse, to the point of near-rudeness. I don't want to know about your holiday or whatever, cut the chit-chat, just let me know why you're phoning. What do you want me to do? Where do you want me to go? My family wouldn't dream of phoning for a chat. I would rather walk ten miles for a chat face to face than answer the phone.

Shortly after I moved to Ireland there was a murder in the Ballymun area of Dublin late one night and, having been informed of the circumstances by Garda Command and Control, I set off to the scene. When I arrived the place was in darkness, with a garda on duty at the front door of the house. He probably thought I was a nosy neighbour or a reporter. When I explained who I was, he told me everyone had gone home and to come back the next morning. I couldn't believe it. Didn't these people know how important it was to start the investigation as soon as possible? That was what the Scottish police always told me.

I turned up the next morning and there was no apology for my aborted visit the night before. When I informed the garda commissioner, he found it hysterically funny that I would be so eager to be at the scene in the middle of the night. On reflection he was quite right, and there is probably more to be lost than gained by blundering about in the dark.

Sometimes my own eagerness worked against me. In one instance the guards wanted me at a scene as soon as possible. I said I'd be there within the hour, depending on traffic. From Swords to Dublin city centre should take twenty minutes or so but at eight in the morning it can take over an hour. That wasn't quick enough so they said they would send a garda escort to get me into town. Great, I thought. A few weeks earlier, travelling down the country to Galway on a bank-holiday weekend I'd got stuck in the traffic on the old N4. After I'd sat in a queue for about thirty minutes, the gardaí sent a car to get me onto the open road. The local guard escorted me past the traffic jam, clearing a path up the middle of the road, with me tucked behind. So, I thought a trip through the streets of Dublin would be a doddle.

Two garda motorbikes arrived at my door and I was told to stick on the tail of the bike at the front and keep all my lights on. I had my doubts, looking at the width of my car and the width of the motorbikes. My one luxury has always been my car. I don't have a social life, no wining and dining or clubbing at the weekend, as I'm usually on call. There is no point in buying expensive clothes as I spend most of my time in the mortuary, so my little indulgence is my transport. I include my shoes in that, my other weakness, but I do need them to get me about, even if they are not practical. I would rather have an older but pretty car than a practical and functional new car, and at that time I had my old Honda Prelude, sleek, low and wide. Very nippy in a straight line, but not designed for weaving in and out of traffic. Isn't that what motorbikes are designed to do? All went well heading down the dual carriageway past the airport. When we got to Whitehall church, the bike behind me drove in front of us into the crossroads to stop the traffic. The bike in front shot forward through the lights, headlights blazing, sirens wailing. I followed at a safe distance.

A big mistake. There is always a driver who will try to squeeze in if you leave any more than a couple of feet between you and the car in front. Panic-stricken, I speeded up and tried to overtake the interloper, but by now I was on the other side of the road. Luckily the lead bike slowed to let me catch up. There was no way I was letting that happen again so I closed the gap between me and the bike in front. He went faster. So did I. All junctions passed in a blur as we raced through town. Finally the bike slowed to a stop when we got to the old city mortuary at Store Street. I was just grateful I'd got there alive. The biker got off and walked over. I was just about to thank him for escorting me when he began jumping up and down and shouting: 'What the hell did you think you were doing?'

I was taken aback. 'I was just following your instructions and trying to keep up with you.' He wasn't impressed with my reasoning. 'Will you be escorting me back?' I enquired. He got back on his bike and left, tyres screeching. I've never accepted an escort since. Thank God, or the EU, for the motorways.

My poor car never recovered from that escapade and a few weeks later blew a gasket. I limped into the car park behind the city mortuary and phoned the AA. I explained that my car had died.

'And where is the car, madam?'

'At the city mortuary.' I thought I'd been cut off. I phoned back but it took some persuading that this wasn't a hoax call.

My first visit to a scene in Glasgow was a few weeks after I'd gone to the dark side and was now a forensic pathologist, albeit in training. The professor thought this might be a good one to start with: it was close to base so if I encountered a problem he could nip over and help. According to the police, it was not likely to be a murder. A young man had been found dead in his home by a relative. He hadn't been seen for a few days.

He was a known drug user. The door had been unlocked. The doctor who had confirmed the death, standard practice, mentioned blood around the body.

It was a foul afternoon, dark and rainy. I found a parking space close to the flats in question and ran up to the close mouth, the opening into the old tenement building. The policeman at the door said, 'Where do you think you're going, hen?'

'I'm Dr Cassidy, blah-blah-blah.'

'Where's the prof?'

I explained that he'd sent me but the policeman said, 'Take my advice, don't go in there, not a sight for a woman!'

I had a job to do so was not to be dissuaded. Reluctantly he let me pass and followed me into the close. He opened the door of the ground-floor flat and stood aside. I was immediately assailed by a smell I had never before experienced. The stench of a decomposing body is an assault to your senses. A lucky few pathologists have no sense of smell. The problem with that, though, is the smell clings to your clothes and your hair: if you don't realise you're giving off the odour of rotting fish, the effect can be very unpleasant for your friends and family.

The smell of decomposition, while something you never forget, is something you can get used to. Forget Vicks on the nostrils and hankies doused in perfume, loved by the police – even masks provide little protection, unless they're heavy duty with their own oxygen supply. Just breathe through your mouth and soon you become accustomed to it. Another good tip is to double-glove and coat the first pair of gloves in very perfumed hand soap. Otherwise when you're eating a sandwich later your hands will be stinking.

On one occasion my colleague and I had examined a badly decomposed body found in a wooded area. The deceased had probably died from drink or natural causes. We finished at lunchtime and decided to stroll over to BHS to do some shopping. He went to the gents department downstairs while I went up to children's wear. I had picked up some nappies and was waiting at the till to pay. A couple of women in the queue in front of me began remarking on an awful smell. It suddenly dawned on me that it was down to me. I dropped the nappies and ran downstairs just as my colleague came rushing towards the exit. In unison we said, 'We smell,' and ran back to the safety of the mortuary.

The smell is a warning at a scene that something very unpleasant is lurking nearby. In the case of my first it should have warned me I was about to meet a very badly decomposed body. The fact that I was not gagging or puking in the corner gave me the courage to cross the room to where it lay. What assailed me was an almost black writhing mass. Getting closer it became obvious that maggots had taken over the body. Although this was my first full-blown putrefying body, I had read the chapter in Professor Ken Masson's book about changes after death and I realised that photographs cannot do this justice.

Ken had written the definitive forensic textbook for lawyers, and his graphic description of the numerous ways to meet an untimely death was probably the main reason most lawyers decided early in their careers that they did not want to be involved in deaths and murders. A few years later I was involved with the special-effects department working on *Taggart*. They had an episode with a decomposed body and wanted to know how to mock it up. I showed them a few photos, getting the usual reaction, 'Oh, that's disgusting!' And that was without the smell. Off they went to produce their version of a decomposing body. A few weeks later they came back to show me the result.

'Oh,' I said. 'That's disgusting!' The production team obviously agreed: when the episode was aired there was only a fleeting glimpse of a blackened foot. That's showbiz.

Back at the scene in Glasgow, the police showed me the 'bloodstaining' that had concerned the doctor who had examined the body, around which there was a brownish puddle of fluid on the linoleum. There was no evidence of any blood elsewhere and, while it was difficult to be sure, there were no obvious injuries on the body. 'Ah!' I said knowingly. 'That's putrefactive fluid. It's part of the postmortem process. The internal organs liquefy and the fluid is purged through the body's orifices. It's not blood from an injury.' With that I turned on my heel and left, desperate to get out of the flat. I hadn't disgraced myself by fainting or any of the normal reactions to witnessing a decaying human. In fact I had a surge of confidence that I could cope with whatever death threw at me.

Back at base I checked my facts before the body and its entourage arrived for the postmortem examination.

The postmortem itself was otherwise uneventful. In other words, I found nothing to account for his death. The toxicology department came up trumps and found heroin in his liver. Phew! Unfortunately, I was to witness many drug-related deaths in Glasgow, such a sad waste of young lives. Most die lonely and alone. At that stage of my career things were black and white. Drug addicts were part of the black. It was after seeing drug addict after drug addict on the mortuary table and visiting the hovels they inhabited that I began to wonder at the power of addiction.

It would be easy to dismiss this group of people and blame the social conditions of their upbringing, the relative poverty in parts of Dublin and Glasgow, for their desire to obliterate their lives, but then I met their families. The majority were ordinary people bewildered by their offspring's choices and devastated by their son or daughter's death. But those deaths were brushed under the carpet in Scotland, not of sufficient public importance to hold any inquiry, so the families mourned in isolation without finding out what had happened and why their son or daughter had died. That's not fair.

The main reason for me to carry out a postmortem is to furnish the family with the result and help them understand what happened. In

Glasgow we set up a Death Clinic. If there was no police investigation into a death, no fatal-accident inquiry – equivalent to a coroner's inquest – and no criminal proceedings, the family was given the opportunity to meet the pathologist. It took just a couple of hours out of my week but the families were grateful that someone was treating them and their deceased relative with respect. Sometimes I was the only person they could discuss the death with, an important part of the process of dealing with it. Another lesson learned along the way.

In Dublin, drug-related deaths are subject to an inquest, which means that the families are privy to the information regarding the cause and circumstances of the death. However, even then, the families in Dublin wanted more than the how or even the why. They have taken a more pragmatic approach and are focusing on damage limitation: arming the vulnerable with the tools to try to prevent unnecessary deaths, striving to get better drug-treatment services. Not for them the patronising platitudes – 'Sorry for your loss. Next' – from those in authority: action is the name of the game. I was lucky enough to witness them in action as part of the group involved in collating the information regarding all deaths in Ireland due to drugs, legal and illegal, and I hope they have the strength to keep going because, without them, there will be a lost tribe in Ireland and we all need to look out for our children.

In Glasgow during the late 1980s and early 1990s, the superintendent in charge always requested the attendance of the pathologist at the scene of a death. Getting information as early as possible in the investigation was, and is, key to a successful outcome, and an expert opinion regarding the cause of death was essential. Before DNA profiling was part of the armour of the forensic scientist, they tended to waft about in a cloud of fingerprint dust, directing the police to collect relevant evidence. There tended to be a more collaborative approach in that era, all chipping in our sixpence worth, more Agatha and Sherlock than Horatio, not Nelson but CSI. Nowadays the forensic scientist is monarch of the scene, and DNA evidence the crown jewels. The rest of us remain loyal subjects but nowadays we have to accept that a pathologist is not going to solve a crime by attending the scene.

There is much to be said about seeing a body *in situ*, particularly if it is a complex scene with multiple sites of bloodstaining and signs of disturbance. Each scene is different, obviously, but, as I've said, from the pathologist's perspective the body is the scene. I like to work backwards from it. Where is the body? Is there blood or evidence of a disturbance around it? Are there obvious injuries, or are injuries obscured by clothing or bloodstaining? How were the injuries caused? Should the police be looking for a blunt object, a knife or gun? Is there blood away from the body? Could the injuries have been inflicted elsewhere? If so, was the victim able to move unaided to where they collapsed or is there evidence to suggest they were dragged to this spot? Often the cause of death is not in question, but the sequence of events may be crucial to the exact circumstances.

Was this a short, swift assault or a prolonged attack? Sometimes there is so much blood at a scene it is difficult to access the body without walking through a pool of it. In these cases foot plates are put down for us to walk on without affecting any potentially crucial evidence. The only problem is that the plates are placed by people who are much taller than I am with a much wider stride. I often have to leap from plate to plate. And, remember, I'm usually doing this in three-inch heels. Ginger Rogers said she did everything Fred Astaire did, but backwards and in heels. Thankfully I don't have to walk backwards. You may think that in thirty-odd years I would have decided to wear 'sensible' shoes, but no.

On one occasion I was called to the scene of death of an elderly male. His body was discovered after his son had phoned the emergency services stating that his father had collapsed. An ambulance arrived but he was already dead. The police were hot on the heels of the paramedics and saw an elderly male slumped in his hall. There appeared to be blood on the wall above and around him, as well as on him and the floor. The son was distraught and told the police he had had an argument with his father during a spot of home decorating and had thrown a tin of paint at him. He was adamant that he hadn't intended to injure his father and was sure the tin hadn't hit him.

I was called to the scene. It wasn't far from the city mortuary so I walked over. I got to the front door and was briefed as to the circumstances. I took one look and turned tail, telling them I had seen enough and to get the body to the mortuary as soon as possible. It was obvious to me that the 'blood' splattered up the wall, in a halo around the old man, was red paint. It took a couple of bottles of turpentine to remove it from the deceased. Just as the son had said, there wasn't a mark on his father. Instead his insides held the explanation. He had a scarred heart due to a previous heart attack. The row with his son over the decorating was enough to tip the balance and cause another. The same would have happened if he'd run for a bus. Still, the son was charged with the manslaughter of his father. I had to give evidence at the trial and, luckily, the jury and the judge were of a mind with me that it would have been very unfair to send the son to prison and he received a suspended sentence.

Copious amounts of blood always cause concern, rightly so. Strange as it may seem, stabbings and shootings can be relatively clean and tidy: death is often so rapid that there is not enough time for the victim to bleed out, their demise being due to damage to the internal organs rather than blood loss. Obviously if the body is left lying for some time blood will seep out of the holes and a pool will form around it. Only if an artery in the neck is severed will blood spurt out at high pressure and spray the surroundings, but cutthroat deaths are relatively uncommon, although the pattern of blood spray – mimicking the rise and fall of the blood pressure curve – is easily recognisable.

In contrast to the often limited and contained blood-staining at the scenes of a stabbing, assaults with a blunt weapon can be incredibly messy, particularly if there are scalp wounds. These incidents are often associated with multiple bleeding lacerations and irregular tears, and the scalp is extremely vascular. Also, death is not usually immediate.

One particular bloody scene catches out police and medics: death after a gastrointestinal haemorrhage. This may be due to a stomach or duodenal ulcer eroding through the wall of the stomach or upper gut and weakening a large artery in the tissues behind. This weakened vessel will eventually rupture, and blood at high force will burst into the stomach and upper gut more quickly than the gut can deal with it. The result is explosive bloody vomiting. When a tumour erodes into an artery the outcome is similar. As an intern, I was called to a ward as someone was vomiting blood. I expected to see the elderly gentleman sitting up in bed with his head in one of those papier-mâché sick bowls. The reality was like something out of *The Exorcist*. He was sitting up in bed spraying bright red arterial blood over everyone and everything within the ward. The nurse looked stricken, I was shocked, but the poor man was obviously terrified. There was nothing I could do – I was as much use as a wet wipe in that situation – but even the surgeon called in couldn't save him. God rest him, what an awful way to go.

A more common scenario in my line of business is the alcoholic with ruptured oesophageal varices. Invariably a man is found dead and there is extensive bloodstaining over and around him. There is a history of chronic alcohol use and, as a result, a rather chequered history, which may have brought him to the attention of the police in the past. Initial examination usually shows bruises on the exposed areas not coated with blood. Such injuries will normally be treated as suspicious until proved otherwise. It's usually an easy case for the pathologist. The blood at the scene is not bright red, not arterial. It isn't even dark purplish venous blood, therefore not from a bleeding injury, but is a brownish red, what we in the trade call 'coffee grounds'. This is blood that has been acted on by acid in the stomach so the source of bleeding must be from that area of the body. Closer inspection will show a yellowish tinge to the skin and the white of the eyes: jaundice.

Aha! I hear you say. Liver damage, alcohol-related cirrhosis. The scarring of the liver affects its blood flow and one of the complications is varicose veins in the oesophagus, knobbly veins jutting into the lumen of the gullet. If these are damaged, they will bleed and the bleeding is difficult to stop. Unfortunately, the seriousness of the situation may not be obvious to the alcoholic and they continue vomiting altered blood until their collapse and death. The pattern of external injuries and the internal findings tell the sad story of self-destruction. Not a murder but another person caught in the web of addiction.

Sometimes the scene can be the cause of death. One young man was found dead in an armchair in his living room. He shared the house with his wife and two children. He had a history of asthma and had been a bit 'chesty' the night before so stayed up after the family went to bed as he felt better sitting upright rather than lying in bed.

It was late on a Friday afternoon by the time I arrived at the small terraced house. It was very neat and tidy, there was no sign of a break-in, no marks on the body, and the man looked as if he had fallen asleep in the chair, a peaceful death, nothing to be concerned about. I agreed that most likely he had had an acute asthmatic attack ... but something about the colour of his face concerned me.

He had a very ruddy complexion. It might have been related to his asthma but similar coloration occurs in those dying from hypothermia and carbon monoxide poisoning. The house was cosy, so it wasn't hypothermia. Carbon monoxide poisoning? Even though everyone thought this was a natural death and the postmortem examination could wait until Monday, I decided to get on with it in case something else cropped up over the weekend. I hate putting deaths on hold. On the way to the mortuary I contacted the toxicologist and asked if he could do an urgent carbon monoxide test.

That would mean staying late on a Friday night, which is never appealing, but eventually he agreed. Another postmortem, another young man with very little to find. Enough changes in the lungs to confirm asthma: a bit over-inflated, mucous plugs in the small airways. But his blood was a definite cherry pink, not diagnostic of carbon monoxide, but an indication. A sample of blood was driven to the laboratory by a disgruntled policeman who should have been at home with the wife and kids. In those days, most detectives were male, but then so were most forensic pathologists.

A couple of hours later I got a panicky call from the toxicologist: there was more than 50 per cent carbon monoxide in the blood, more than enough to kill someone with damaged lungs. Instead of relief that I had been right, it was my turn to panic. We had left a young family in a dangerous situation, probably with many more arriving to offer their condolences. If we didn't act quickly we could be dealing with many more deaths.

Luckily the police were still in the mortuary finishing off. Although they were initially reluctant to rush over and throw everyone out of the house, a quick chat with the toxicologist made them realise the seriousness of the situation. It transpired that the deceased had put in a new gas boiler, not very well as it was not his trade, and had also fitted super-duper double-glazing. That fateful night, as he was staying up late and it was a little chilly, he had put on the heating for the first time.

The case showed the danger of not using properly qualified professionals when doing work on your house. What price do you place on your and your family's lives?

Generally, the first policeman at the scene of a death has to decide whether or not it is to be treated as 'suspicious'. In the majority of cases the decision is straightforward, signalled by massive amounts of blood, horrendous injuries or evidence of a struggle. But sometimes it's more of a feeling that something is not quite right. These are usually the more interesting scenes. One such case started as a possible suicide.

The death of Siobhan Kearney, in 2006, presented as an Agatha Christie mystery: woman discovered dead in a locked bedroom. Her young child had been found alone in the house by a relative, who guessed that Siobhan was in the locked bedroom and that something must be badly wrong. Other family members rushed to the house and managed to force the door open. They found Siobhan dead on the floor. There was a mark on her neck and the flex of a vacuum cleaner fashioned into a noose beside her. The initial thought was that this was a sad suicide, and she had locked her bedroom door so the child wouldn't find her. But when the gardaí arrived they thought it was rather unusual. When the senior investigating officer phoned me, he said, 'It just doesn't feel right.' That piqued my interest.

Off I went. The house, unusually, was in a very nice area. I was ushered upstairs and immediately could see what the issue was. The scene was as it had been described to me, but I agreed that it just wasn't right. Watching where I was treading, I entered the bedroom. On the floor, near to the door, there was a key and a photograph. Facing me was the bed. The covers were crumpled, more than I would have expected even for someone who had had a restless night contemplating taking their own life. The room was large, and a few feet from the bottom of the bed, a blonde-haired woman clad in a jumper and pyjama bottoms lay face up on the floor.

The most striking feature was her deep red face, partly due to a mass of small pinpoint haemorrhages covering it. There was a mark across her neck and some grazes on her chin. I had no doubt that her death was due to asphyxia, a lack of oxygen as a result of her neck being compressed. The mark on her neck suggested that a ligature had squeezed the vessels in her neck, restricting the blood flow through the jugular veins causing the pressure to build up in the small capillaries under the skin until they ruptured, causing the ruddy appearance.

I was assured that no one had moved the body and that this was the exact position in which she had been found. She was lying in the right-hand corner at the far end of the room, away from the bedroom door. Close to the body was a vacuum cleaner, the flex coiled and knotted, forming a noose of sorts. There were mirrored wardrobes behind her head and the door to the en-suite was to her right side. She wasn't particularly close to either. There was no evidence of a ligature attached to a suspension point, such as the doors, which is what I would expect at the scene of a hanging, and the 'noose' was beside her and not around her neck. Odd.

I have examined the scenes of many deaths due to hanging. Generally, people choose a fairly robust material and the majority are still hanging when their bodies are found. Sometimes the ligature fails and snaps, leaving part still attached to the suspension point and the noose still around the neck, the person in a crumpled heap immediately below the point of suspension. On occasion the ligature ruptures immediately it takes the strain, and the person drops to the ground. In this instance, things didn't add up.

There were many aspects which troubled me, from her position to the marks and injuries on her neck and face. Had this been a suicidal hanging, I would have expected her to be still suspended when found, and the point of suspension to be obvious. There was a ligature mark on Siobhan's neck but the ligature was not around her neck. In full-suspension hanging, the ligature takes the full weight of the body and death occurs rapidly, and while there will be a ligature mark on the neck, the face is pale. There were also other marks on her face which couldn't be accounted for.

So, I had my concerns that this scene had either been disturbed by those finding the body, who didn't want to admit it, or the scene had been staged to look like a suicidal hanging. I favoured the latter. I was leaning towards this being a homicide and that Siobhan had been strangled with a ligature. The state of the bed suggested she had been attacked while in bed, perhaps even sleeping, and that she had struggled with her attacker on the bed. The gardaí were concerned that the position of the key on the floor didn't fit with it having fallen from the keyhole on the inside of the door after she had locked it. Its proximity to the photograph on the floor made them wonder if the door had been locked from the outside and the key slid under it. These incongruities are what make a death 'suspicious'.

But a feeling in your water doesn't stand up in court, so if you have a theory you have to prove it. The pathologist in this instance can take the case only so far: the postmortem findings were highly suggestive of ligature strangulation by a third party rather than hanging. The injuries to her neck, in particular the damage to her Adam's apple, were more severe and extensive than would be expected in a suicidal hanging. But 'suggestive' is not definitive proof. Could there be an alternative, less sinister, explanation for the marks on her neck and face? Might she have been part-suspended? Perhaps she had attached the ligature to a suspension point that meant her feet were touching the floor: however, while this would make it less likely that the ligature would break, it might explain her ruddy complexion – death in this type of hanging is not as rapid as it is in full suspension. But it would not explain the other marks on her face. Also, despite denials of moving her body, someone might have moved her just enough to be able to examine her properly.

Did the evidence at the scene support suicide or murder?

Only the forensic scientists could take the investigation to the next stage. Assuming that this was a self-inflicted hanging, the scientists attempted to reconstruct the possible scenarios that would result in Siobhan's death and explain her position at the scene. The scene was scoured for evidence of a potential suspension point, of which there was none. In the forensic science laboratory, the vacuum flex was tested to determine not only if it could support Siobhan's weight – it could – but also the load required to cause the flex to fail and snap.

Her position when found could not be accounted for. It was painstaking work but eventually the evidence came together. Pathologist and scientists were in agreement: this was not suicide. The DPP agreed there was sufficient evidence to support that this was a murder, with the husband as prime suspect. The forensic scientists reconstructed their experiments in court to explain how the hanging theory did not stand up to scrutiny. That, with the postmortem findings, led the jurors to convict Siobhan's husband of murder.

Ireland is unusual in that there is a culture of concealing bodies. In Scotland, concealment meant pulling the covers over the body or putting it into a bin or, in one instance, dropping the body through a manhole into the sewage system. The latter was a rather unusual case. A body was discovered in a water treatment plant near Glasgow. Strangely this was the second body to turn up there. The previous one had been a shooting with quick disposal of the body and, once discovered, rapid identification of the victim. This one, though, was more of a problem.

In Scotland, as I've said, two pathologists are involved in the investigation of a suspicious death. This ensures that there is little chance of getting things wrong, but it's not fool-proof. Only one of the two needs to attend the scene, as long as both are present at the postmortem. With this in mind, I sent my deputy to the scene, with the advice to take a pair of wellingtons and a change of clothing. Sewage smells. It was obvious from the position of the body that it had not just been dumped into the open tank at the sewage works but had had to travel through the sewage system to end up where it was. While the police set out to work on that, the body was brought to the mortuary for examination.

This was a male, fully clothed. He had obviously been dead for some weeks as there was evidence of advanced decomposition. The head was deformed, probably indicating death due to head trauma, although we were unsure what damage would be done to a body on its passage through the sewage system. There were gaping holes on either side of the trunk, and the internal organs were largely missing. The skin remaining on the front of the chest was scorched, indicating contact with flame and possible attempts to get rid of the body by burning. Even more sinister, the hands were missing, not just detached as part of decomposition, which can happen: they had been crudely chopped off mid-forearm. No hands, no fingers, no fingerprints. Someone didn't want us to know who the man was. The linchpin to any murder investigation is knowing who the victim was because that will lead the police to the perpetrator.

The working hypothesis was that this man had been the victim of an assault causing fatal head trauma and there had been a deliberate attempt to conceal the crime by disposing of the body.

The postmortem examination confirmed that death was due to head trauma, the skull was fragmented and the brain was now partly liquified. Due to the postmortem changes, natural and inflicted, there was little to assist us in identification or determining the circumstances of the death, otherwise.

There was rope around the body, but this might just have become entangled with it in the sewage system. The clothing was high-end high street and the shoes were fashionable leather lace-ups. This was obviously someone with a bit of money: surely someone was missing him. In an effort to identify him I called on our forensic dentist to chart the teeth in the hope that if police enquiries provided a tentative identity we would be able to access that person's dental records for comparison with the deceased's dentition.

Meanwhile the police had had much fun dropping plastic canisters into the sewage system in various locations trying to pin down where he had gone into the drain system. What this experiment revealed was that, once it was in the system, a canister arrived at the sewage plant within twenty-four hours. That didn't fit with our belief that the man had been dead for weeks. Where had the body been kept after death before it got into the sewage system?

About this time a woman came forward to report her husband, George Hall, missing. They had been at a karaoke night in a local pub several weeks prior to this. She had gone to the toilet, and when she'd come back he had disappeared.

She hadn't seen him since and thought she should report him missing. Could this have something to do with the newspaper reports of a body being found? Could this be our body? Armed with the name, the police tried to find his dentist to get his dental records.

They also went to the pub to make some enquiries, only to find it had been partly destroyed in a recent fire. The owner was unable to assist them. Over the next few days the police tracked down some people who had been in the pub the night George Hall had gone missing. One man said he remembered a couple sitting opposite him: at one point the man was sitting on his own, there was a whooshing noise, then the man collapsed and vomited reddish fluid. Suddenly two men appeared from the kitchen area, rushed over, lifted the man and took him out. A short time later the woman came back to the table, picked up her things and left. Was this our man? Unfortunately, the forensic dentist had gone away for a few days after he had examined the body but I asked if he could deal with this as a matter of urgency to see if we could get a positive ID. The police brought George Hall's dental records to the dentist and he confirmed they were a match. The body was George Hall.

I began thinking about the eyewitness's account. A whooshing noise followed by collapse. Could he have been shot? There were no X-ray facilities in the mortuary but there were in the dental hospital. Although the dental hospital was more used to live patients, they agreed to assist us in this instance. X-rays showed a deformed bullet lodged in the upper cervical spine. Bingo. We had a cause of death.

But how did it fit together? The detectives, ballistics experts and I went to the burned-out pub to try to reconstruct the scene. We knew the seating arrangement of the relevant parties. The kitchen was the only vantage point for a gunman to remain out of view of the customers. George and his wife had been seated directly facing the kitchen. Seated where he was, if George was shot at from the kitchen, the bullet would have struck his chest, not his head or neck. This meant that the gunshot to the head happened later after he had been removed from the pub. Likely the chest injury had wounded but not killed him and he was finished off with a shot to the head. Surprisingly, despite the lapse of time and the recent fire damage to the pub, a bucket and mop found in the kitchen had traces of George's blood. That forensic evidence put him at the scene.

The only conundrum was, how had the body ended up in the sewage works several weeks later? Information filtered down to the police that a man and his wife had been in that same pub a couple of nights before the pub fire, regaling the customers with the tale of her husband coming across a body. She held the floor as she told of how he had set off to a local wooded area with a washing line intending to hang himself. The trees, though, were mostly saplings, which wouldn't have taken his weight. With a sudden flash of inspiration, he came up with the idea of attaching the rope to a tree trunk, then jumping down into the drainage system. He lifted the manhole cover and, not surprisingly, was shocked to see a body on a ledge a few feet below. He raced home and told his wife. Presumably in an effort to cheer him up, she suggested going out for a drink, possibly not the recommended treatment for depression. It is likely that one of those involved in George's death was in their audience and raced off to check this out for himself. Imagine his shock at seeing George perched on the ledge. There was no option but to climb down to the ledge and push the body into the vortex below. Hours later George popped up in the water treatment works.

It transpired that a friend of the deceased's wife was the culprit and at trial he was found guilty of murder. Sometimes they try too hard to disguise their crimes.

In Ireland we often had to look harder to find a body. This often included some expert digging by anthropologists. Of course, the most notorious cases are those who went missing, presumed dead, during the Troubles in Northern Ireland, the 'Disappeared'.

Most people can't deal with the death of a loved one until they see the proof. There is always a tiny bit of hope that the missing person just disappeared and is alive and well somewhere else. It is difficult to grieve or move on until you know the truth. So, even if it's not what we think we would want, it is a huge relief to families to know for certain what happened, then be allowed to have a funeral and at last have others acknowledge the death. I cannot imagine how families desperate for news must feel each time a search begins and is unsuccessful. At the start of each one the hopes are high but in some cases, after months of excavation of a particular area, a decision has to be made to abandon the attempt. That must be heartbreaking for the relatives.

'Thou art dust and into dust you shall return,' but first you have to go through the process of decomposition and decay. After months or years, depending on where a body lies, it will be skeletalised, reduced to bare bones. That presents two problems to the pathologist: determining the cause of death and identifying the remains. The wise pathologist enlists the assistance of a forensic anthropologist, a specialist in examining bones, old and modern. Working together, the pathologist and anthropologist will ensure the optimum information is gleaned.

In Ireland Laureen Buckley is the most experienced forensic anthropologist, usually to be found in the bowels of the museum in the company of ancient remains, way older than me and 'my' remains.

Once it was established that a body of one of the missing 'Disappeared' had been uncovered, Laureen and I would normally attend the site and assist the anthropologists in the removal of the body. In some instances the family had maintained a vigil throughout the excavation. After all that time the main issue was identification of the remains. In 1999 the Independent Commission for the Location of Victims' Remains was set up as part of a treaty between the UK and Ireland. It was responsible for the search and recovery of the remains of sixteen missing persons. There would be no investigation into the circumstances of the deaths; the remains would be identified and returned to the family. I immediately agreed to be part of the team involved.

Luckily, the families of those missing had been able to give the Commission detailed descriptions of clothing and distinguishing features. Despite being hampered by the distorting effect of decomposition, the information provided was sufficient for us to be pretty sure we had the correct body. The general postmortem examination was always followed by DNA analysis, the scientific proof of identity. Another body rightfully returned to its family.

Burial is one way to get rid of the evidence. Another is fire. It is very difficult to destroy a body by fire without a great deal of effort – even crematoria find it a challenge. Bodies are extremely robust. Skin is our protective layer and is fairly water and fire resistant. It may smoulder but won't normally flame. 'Spontaneous human combustion' is recognised as a condition by forensic pathologists. Of course it is a complete misnomer – no one simply erupts into flame – but the scene is so unusual that these deaths are often treated as suspicious, as are those where bodies are recovered from a house or building fire.

Strangely enough, despite the extent of destruction of the body by fire, forensic pathologists can usually get to the bottom of such a death. In spontaneous human combustion there are key findings. Fire damage is localised to the area around the body, there is a source of ignition, and often the deceased has been drinking. Commonly the source of the fire is a dropped lit cigarette but it might be a spark from a hearth or an electrical fault. Such scenes have to be examined by fire experts.

The body itself shows extensive burns to perhaps the upper or lower half, the rest of the body a little soot-stained but relatively spared the effect of heat. The unusual appearance is due to the property of the body tissues. The fire, once it takes hold, causes smouldering of the skin and underlying fatty tissue. If the person has been drinking, alcohol present in the fatty tissue fuels the fire and allows it to continue burning and not burn itself out. It's a diagnosis that can be made at the scene.

There is always concern that a fire has been used to conceal a homicide. That does happen, but the pathologist can usually determine whether or not the person was dead before the fire started, looking for soot in the airways and high levels of carbon monoxide in the blood. Only if the body is completely reduced to ashes can there be a problem.

In 2003, Dolores McRea was reported missing by her sister, and the police began making enquiries, trying to establish when and where she was last seen alive. One of the people questioned was her ex-husband. According to the family, she was intending to visit him. When the police arrived at his door a bonfire was blazing in the garden. It looked like he was burning tyres and other materials. However, on closer inspection a policeman thought he saw a human thigh bone in the middle of the flames. A local doctor was brought to the scene and he agreed. Was this our missing woman? The ex-husband assured the police that the bones were animal but an investigation was launched.

I was called to the scene, as were the forensic team, but we had to travel from Dublin to Donegal, and the fire raged on. To expedite matters the gardaí arranged to transport me to the scene. I naively assumed that the fire would be extinguished by the time the forensic team arrived, but that wasn't to be. I knew that this was obviously going to be a difficult case and did not want to do anything to scupper the investigation.

Before the Technical Bureau waded in I called the forensic anthropologist Laureen Buckley for advice. I asked what would be the effect on bones if we tried to extinguish the fire. Water would fragment any large pieces, I was told. So we tried a powder fire extinguisher, but the fire continued burning. If we were to recover any valuable material we needed to get into the fire before all we had was a pile of ash. Not ideal conditions but we had no option. We had to pick through the hot embers as best we could. Most of us had burned fingertips but nothing was going to stop us trying to recover as much as was humanly possible. Interestingly, a metal bed frame had been in the fire and provided us with a makeshift grid, which we used to plot out the position of the small fragments we collected. That was to prove invaluable. There were a few large pieces, a few centimetres across, which were obviously bone, and some small fragments of burned bone identifiable. Hours later, we and the fire were exhausted. Several trays of fire debris were taken back to Dublin for anthropological examination.

I left Laureen in the mortuary in Dublin to do her magic, and that she did. From the charred debris a skeletal outline emerged, the phoenix rising from the ashes. Not only was there sufficient to confirm these were human remains but they were the remains of a female. I had even found numerous teeth, which were instrumental in her identification. The slender bone from the neck, part of the Adam's apple, was present and this was damaged, raising the possibility that she hadn't accidentally fallen into a bonfire but was killed and the bonfire was an attempt to cover that up.

Beware, your sins will find you out.

4

Identification

A BODY WAS FOUND IN a skip in Glasgow. The man had been brutally assaulted, and even peering over the side into the depths of the skip it was clear that his death was due to a severe head injury. Brain tissue was smudged over the inside of the skip. The body was taken to the city mortuary where it became apparent that this had been a savage assault and, importantly, there had been extreme attempts to prevent identification of the deceased. There were no possessions to give any clue as to who he was, the face was badly disfigured, the teeth deliberately damaged, and the fingers had been amputated.

That left DNA. But DNA would be useful

only if we had an idea of who the man might be. This is a constant problem with dental and DNA identification methods. Even a DNA database can take us only so far.

Among the myriad of injuries, there was a mark on his arm that I thought might be from a bite. The area was swabbed in case the perpetrator had transferred saliva to the victim, which might be useful in identifying the person responsible. Could we solve the case by finding the killer's identity and hoping that led to the deceased's? Forensic pathologists are not experts in dental identification so I contacted our dental expert, Professor McDonald from the dental hospital, for assistance.

While he examined the possible bite mark on the body, the mortuary team – myself, the technicians and the police – left him to it and had a cup of tea in the mortuary office. We weren't expecting much. I had explained to him that the teeth were in bits or missing so we didn't think he would be able to assist in identifying the owner. However, when he came out of the mortuary, he told me the injury on the arm wasn't a bite mark but he thought he might be able to identify the deceased.

Wow! What a coincidence! Who would have

thought he'd treated the man? 'Oh, no, I've never seen him before. But among the fragments of broken teeth you collected there was part of a broken upper denture and someone has scratched a name on it. It's either his or that of the technician who made the plate.'

A vital piece of evidence. It was the name of the deceased. Body identified. Now the police could try to track his murderer. Since then I always have a good look at dental plates before I summon a dentist's assistance to identify a John Doe.

Knowing the identity of the deceased person is crucial to any death investigation. It may assist in providing a motive for a murder, reveal a psychiatric disorder pointing to suicide, or a medical history that may be the reason for a sudden unexplained death. Every Jane or John Doe deserves to be identified and returned to their family.

This is not a problem in the majority of deaths. Most deaths are due to natural causes and people die in their own home or after admission to hospital, often with their nearest and dearest around them, or their body is discovered by someone close to them. Grandparents, mothers, fathers, siblings and, sadly, children usually have someone who loves them and can confirm who they were. They are the fortunate ones. If the body is undamaged and they are recently dead, nothing more than viewing it at home, or in an institution, is required to confirm the identity of the deceased. This applies to the majority of those dying from natural causes. When there is no immediate family, the patient's GP may be able to identify the person when they arrive to confirm death, a process required in all deaths.

If the death has been reported to the coroner for further investigation, there is a legal requirement for someone related to the deceased, or someone who has known them for some time, to formally identify the body, even if they were the person who reported the death or were in the house when the police or gardaí arrived. This entails visiting the mortuary and identifying the body to the police or gardaí. Quite traumatic, but every effort is made to ensure that it is as painless as possible. But it must be done. The identity is simply confirmed by facial identification.

Depending on the mortuary, the family may be brought into a room with a glass screen, on the other side of which is the covered body, or there may be a monitor with the image of the deceased's face. The family are asked whether they recognise this person and, if so, to give the deceased's full name. In some hospitals the family will be brought into the room where the body lies. If the death is being treated as a potential homicide they will not be allowed to touch it.

Facial identification is quick and satisfactory in the majority of cases, but it is subjective and mistakes can be made. Sometimes people don't want to accept the death and are adamant that this body is not their family member. In some instances it may occur because the deceased is not wearing their spectacles or we've combed their hair to the wrong side. On one occasion an elderly man was brought into the mortuary to identify his wife. He looked at the image on the screen, his head bobbing from side to side, trying to see the face from a different angle. After a few minutes he admitted he wasn't sure. 'Can you show me her feet?' The mortuary technician was sent to change the angle of the camera. Up popped the feet on the screen. 'Aye, that's her. I've looked after those corns for years.'

Unfortunately some people die alone or in circumstances where identification cannot be assumed or determined immediately: those with no family or friends, the person nipping out for a pint of milk with nothing but money in their pocket and collapsing in the street or even being mown down by a car. Then there are those disfigured by trauma, fire or the effects of decomposition, and bodies removed from rivers or the sea. We may assume that the incinerated remains in a house fire are those of the person last known to be living at that address or that the body found dead in the hotel room is who he or she said they were when they checked in, but how can we be sure? The deceased may have identifying papers on them but those on their own are not reliable.

If there is a chance that the body could be identified visually, if someone who knows them is found, one approach is to provide the investigating authorities with a full description of the personal characteristics of the deceased: sex, approximate age, race, height, weight, hair length, style and colour, eye colour, any distinguishing features, moles, scars, tattoos, deformities, jewellery and the clothing worn. This may be sufficient to allow the police to approach a family to make general enquiries and try to confirm that the deceased is the person named on the bank card that was in their pocket or bag. The family will then be invited to accompany the police to the mortuary to view and formally identify the body. This prevents a family being unnecessarily traumatised by being informed of a death in error. Although the system is not fool-proof.

On one occasion the body of a young man was found on waste ground. He had died of a drug overdose. Papers in his possession identified him as an American citizen. Police enquiries led them to an aunt with whom he had been staying while on holiday. She had not seen him for some days and it was assumed that her nephew and the young man in the mortuary were one and the same. She was escorted to the mortuary and confirmed that this was her nephew. She had to inform his parents and was extremely upset that this had happened while he was visiting her. The family back home asked for the body to be returned.

This involved special arrangements, including an agreement from the procurator fiscal that the body could be embalmed, placed in a coffin and removed from Scotland. The body arrived in America and arrangements were made for the family to view it. When the coffin was opened, to the parents' consternation the body inside was not their son's. At first it was thought that a mistake had been made at the Glasgow end and that the wrong body had been dispatched. It was returned.

Meanwhile the 'deceased' had turned up alive and well, having taken off for a tour around Scotland. Before he left Glasgow he had 'lost' a bag which must have contained an ID card, not worth bothering about as he still had his wallet and bank cards. Aunt was relieved, but shamefaced at having wrongly identified the dead man as her nephew. This was before the era of the mobile phone, which is useful for keeping in touch and informing family of your whereabouts (but, remember, it is keeping tabs on you). In this instance, all ended well for one family, but the real deceased was never identified, no known loving family looking for him.

If there are no accompanying personal belongings, the police may release the description of an unidentified body to the media in the hope that the family will come forward or someone may have information as to the events that led up to the person's death. This is the reverse process of when a person is reported missing: then the family is asked to provide the description of them. Not as easy as it would seem. I often ask my students to describe the person on one side of them without looking at him or her. Taking into consideration that these students have spent the best part of four years together, and only a few moments before I started my lecture they had all been having important conversations with one another, they find it difficult to give an accurate description of their neighbour.

Try it yourself: you may be able to describe their general features, but accurate heights and weights are difficult, and describing the clothing someone was wearing when they left the house can be particularly tricky as most of us are distracted or not very alert first thing in the morning.

If the body fails to be identified by these means, or cannot be identified by facial recognition, due to trauma, advanced decomposition or the effects of fire or water, we will employ scientific methods, principally fingerprints, dental comparison and DNA, but radiology may also be useful. The drawback with these methods is that we need a reference point – in other words, some idea of who the body is to confirm its identity.

Fingerprints are unchanging and unique, but not durable, which is unfortunate as this precludes their use in identifying bodies damaged in fires, decomposed bodies, and bodies removed from water after being immersed for enough time for the skin to start detaching from the hands. Identification by the fingerprint method requires the fingerprints and palm prints to be taken from the body. These are known as latent prints and are compared with prints from another source, either a database of prints deliberately taken from known persons, or prints taken from objects handled by the deceased. The major problem with this method of identification is that only a small percentage of a population's fingerprints is on file. The majority are those of criminals whose fingerprints are stored on a police database, but others include merchant seamen and airline pilots, people at significant risk of dying during the course of their employment.

Despite the drawback, during the course of a homicide postmortem the body will be fingerprinted. The prints are useful in identifying an unknown only if that person has a criminal record and their prints are on the police database, or if the deceased was the target in a gangland killing or it was a drug-related death.

In the past, comparing the latent prints from a body with deliberately taken fingerprints, either stored on a database or lifted from objects, was a manual process. The fingerprints experts would compare and contrast the prints using a points system, looking for similarities. There had to be several points of comparison, the exact number varying from jurisdiction to jurisdiction, but between eight and sixteen. This is largely subjective and the reliability of the results depended on the quality of the latent print and the skill, training and experience of the fingerprint examiner. There was always the possibility of human error and cases of mistaken identity.

Over the last couple of decades, with the introduction of comprehensive computerised police databases, the process is now largely automated. AFIS, Automated Fingerprint Identification Systems, have been developed to analyse the latent prints and generate potential 'candidates', which are further scrutinised by human fingerprint experts. The end result will be a positive, or negative, identification, but in some instances the result will be inconclusive. The reliability of this evidence depends on the quality and uniqueness of the print.

In the past there has been criticism of fingerprint methods. In 1989, in London, the *Marchioness*, a party vessel, went down in the Thames. Fifty-one young people died. It took some days to recover all the bodies and the longer they were in the water the more difficult the process of identification became. A decision was made by the coroner to identify the bodies by taking their fingerprints and comparing them with prints lifted from personal items recovered from the homes of those presumed dead. Taking fingerprints from deteriorating bodies proved difficult so a decision was made to cut off the hands of about half of the bodies and take them to the laboratory for printing. The hands were to be sewn back on to the bodies before they were released for disposal by the family. Unfortunately, not all the hands were returned and families only became aware of that at the inquest some considerable time later. They were extremely angered. Forensic pathologists usually try not to mutilate bodies but at that time the method employed was fairly commonplace.

Thankfully, techniques have improved and this is something we would not contemplate today. Most fingerprint experts have developed techniques to enable them to print even badly decomposed bodies. In Dublin, this was highlighted by the Garda fingerprinter Mick, who managed to fingerprint a 'bog body', proving that even thousands of years after death anything is possible.

Dental identification, comparing the teeth of the deceased with their dental records, proves more useful than fingerprints in situations such as fire deaths and decomposition, but dental work is not necessarily unique. This method requires the expertise of a forensic dentist to chart the restorations and anomalies of the teeth of an unidentified body. Unfortunately, it is not as simple as charting the teeth of the deceased and running the results through a national computer database. There is no such thing.

Again, we need to have some idea as to who the deceased was, then ascertain who was their dentist. Does your family know who your dentist is? When you last visited your dentist, did he or she chart your teeth? Not all do, and even if they did, mistakes are easily made and sometimes the chart is not entirely accurate. Some dentists chart only the work they do. How many different dentists have you visited? Even with all the relevant information the forensic dentist will not definitively identify a body, but rather he or she will opine that the evidence is not inconsistent with the body being a particular individual. If the dentition is unique, or if there are dental X-rays available, the forensic dentist may be able to be more definitive.

A problem we encountered in Ireland was that

some individuals with a medical card, entitling them to free dental care, would occasionally help a family member or friend by lending them their card. This caused confusion when the owner of the card came to a sticky end. To identify them we resorted to dentistry but when their teeth were compared to 'their' dental records there was a mismatch. There was less work done than recorded in the records, fewer fillings, and teeth were present that were recorded as removed. A sensitive discussion with the family will usually resolve the situation. They will come clean if it is explained that the inconsistencies prevent the body being identified and therefore it cannot be returned to them.

In some cases, identification of the body is more important than how the person met his or her death. This is the case in conflicts. We know the young men and women who went off to war. We know the cause of death of most of them. But families want their loved ones back. In the late 1980s, long before I got involved with the United Nations, I met an American anthropologist at a forensic meeting in Australia. Our professor was supposed to go but became unwell. It was all paid for so I was asked if I fancied going in his place. Hell, yes. Whenever was I going to get another chance like that?

Only a few from the UK were attending the conference, including our senior toxicologist and a couple of forensic physicians. We clung together like castaways and picked up other waifs and strays along the way. One was a forensic anthropologist. She worked for the American government and was based in Hawaii. Her role was to assist in recovering the remains of all American servicemen dying in conflicts overseas. Little did I know then that a few years later I would be doing similar work, assisting in the identification of bodies in mass graves.

1990s Glasgow was a busy time for the forensic department. In 1992, there were ninety-two homicides. That's about two per week. I saw more of my forensic colleagues than I did of my family. I was vaguely aware of a war in Yugoslavia but, like everyone else, I had more than enough to worry about back home, juggling work and the family. I was dealing with murders, suicides and accidents, enough death without having to worry about people dying abroad. It's always somebody else's problem . . . until it's not.

Professor Watson retired and a Professor Vanesis was appointed. He had worked in London and was involved with the British military forces providing forensic services for soldiers dying abroad. When a soldier dies abroad there still has to be an inquiry into the death. Relatively few were killed in conflict at that time but some died in road traffic accidents and tragically some committed suicide. As if we hadn't enough to do in Glasgow, suddenly we were running a world-wide service. I had a few trips to Germany, where there was a large military presence following the Second World War, which were a bit more exciting than visiting a scene in Maryhill.

Professor Vanesis was also involved in an organisation called Physicians for Human Rights. I was aware of them but assumed they dealt with live victims in war zones and such, which they did, but under the auspices of the United Nations they became involved in investigating allegations of war crimes on a phenomenal scale in Rwanda and former Yugoslavia. Suddenly those wars became our business. I was reminded of the conversations I had had with the American forensic anthropologist in Australia about the recovery of American soldiers' bodies in areas of conflict, and I immediately agreed to get involved.

I'm not political. I have a simplistic approach to death: it needs to be investigated, and if there is evidence that the death was unlawful, steps should be taken to provide justice for the deceased. And that means going through the correct channels. I am not a vigilante and it is not for me to decide who is right or wrong: there are always two sides to the story. I can bring only my expertise to the table and present my findings in an unbiased factual manner, whether I am dealing with one body, hundreds or thousands.

My first trip was to Tuzla, Bosnia, in 1996, where an international team of forensic pathologists was investigating the mass graves that were being discovered in the aftermath of the war. I flew into Zagreb, in Croatia and also part of the former Yugoslavia, and was collected at the airport and taken to the UN headquarters. There was only one tiny problem: my luggage didn't turn up. Unfortunately, due to the nature of my journey, I couldn't get travel insurance although, knowing I would spend my days in a makeshift mortuary and live in basic accommodation, I had nothing of value and had been informed that any clothing I brought would probably best be left behind. I was assured that my bag would turn up the next day and we would continue our journey across country to Tuzla. The next day it had not turned up, but the UN had much more pressing business than worrying about a stray bag so it was decided that everyone would head off as planned in the jeeps and I would follow on a bus with my bag.

I was given a piece of paper with the details of where to catch the bus and where I was to be dropped off, but the instructions were written in a language I didn't understand. I wasn't happy about this but didn't want to make a fuss, so I waved them off and waited. The bag did not appear and I had no option but to get the bus the next day. I had no idea where I was going or how far it was. I just hoped the driver would remember to let me know when we got there. It took the best part of a day and I was so relieved when I saw one of the UN personnel waiting for me at the bus stop in Tuzla.

Pathologists from the UK, the USA and Europe were involved in the mission with the International Criminal Tribunal over the next few years. Most of us could manage only a couple of weeks at a time, taking holidays from our work back home. In Tuzla a group of Americans was in residence, including a couple of pathologists, numerous anthropologists and police. The visiting pathologists were expected to parachute in and continue the examination of bodies found in mass graves.

The work was sensitive, and there was ill feeling towards the UN mission in that area of the country, the local people wary of our involvement, so we needed protection at all times at the mortuary and travelling to and from it. On a couple of occasions the minibus and jeeps were ambushed, but luckily there were no casualties. The mortuary was an old textile factory that had been badly damaged during the war. There was a generator supplying electricity, but only to the refrigerated units containing the bodies and an area with X-ray equipment. There was no running water. Trestle tables were set up as work stations for us.

Everything was rudimentary. A toilet and shower block had been erected but there was a limited supply of hot water, as the tank had to be refilled by army personnel bringing in water from their base. We were instructed that we should flush only when necessary, and when showering at the end of the day, we should turn the shower on to get wet, turn it off, soap up, and rinse for as short a time as possible. We British were very good at following these instructions, but others weren't, so I often had cold showers.

The mortuary was outside the main town and we were warned not to stray into the grounds as there were landmines, and possibly snipers in the area. There were no facilities to prepare food so we lived on military rations, MREs. Our living conditions weren't much better. We were staying in two houses, sharing rooms. The town had been badly hit during the war and the buildings bore the scars. There was hot water for one hour in the morning. It was unpredictable as to when it would kick in, and once we heard the pipes gurgling there would be a stampede to get in for a hot shower, particularly if you'd missed your chance the night before at the mortuary. So, it wasn't a luxury trip.

But nothing could have prepared us for the work we faced. Walking towards the dilapidated building, the stench from the mortuary was overpowering and, due to lack of washing facilities, we smelt of rotting corpses for the whole time we were there. The missing suitcase didn't appear until two days before I was due to leave. I had no option but to borrow clothes from the others, who were mostly big beefy Americans. I looked like a refugee. Even a trip to the military base, which had a small shop, wasn't too helpful, but at least I got a few pairs of boxer shorts, even though they were size XXL. The army doesn't cater for five-foot weaklings.

Outside the mortuary were the refrigerated

trucks where the bodies excavated from mass graves were stored, awaiting examination. By the time I had arrived the anthropologists had excavated two mass graves. This is a painstaking process: it took months to discover the hidden graves and weeks to uncover the bodies. It requires meticulous precision: those bodies were more important to us than any artefact recovered from the Pyramids, and their recovery requires time and patience, anthropologists with trowels and paintbrushes, not pathologists with spades.

Excavation was difficult, the level of difficulty depending on whether it was a primary grave, where the bodies were interred immediately after death, or the tangled remains of a secondary or tertiary grave. In those cases the bodies have been moved to another location to prevent their discovery, during which process the primary grave will have been churned up by a digger, scooping up the bodies and dumping them, higgledy-piggledy, in a large hole somewhere distant from the original grave, then covering it. The anthropologists dig a trench around the suspected site to define the boundary of the mound of bodies, then slowly uncover the remains, piled one upon another.

As a body, body part or artefact is uncovered,

a universal standard system is used and each and every piece of evidence is given a unique identifying number. Once the anthropologists are satisfied that they have numbered each body, body part or artefact *in situ*, the individually numbered remains are put into separate body bags, again bearing the unique identifying number. The bags are transported to a storage area, which may be a refrigerated truck, and taken in turn to the mortuary to await examination. In Tuzla the resources were limited so the bodies were piled high, one on top of another, inside the refrigerated containers. It was disturbing to see when you opened the door for the first time, but necessary to try to preserve the bodies as best we could in order to get from them the required information. In general, the more deteriorated the body, the more difficult it is to identify the deceased and determine the cause of death. The process is exactly the same whether dealing with a stabbing in Glasgow, a shooting in Dublin or a mass grave in former Yugoslavia.

In the early phase of recovery of bodies from the mass graves in former Yugoslavia, the emphasis was on proving that these deaths were war crimes. The numbers were so overwhelming that we thought we would never be able to identify all the remains recovered. We were aware that we had to make sure that we noted anything about the body or on it that in the future might lead to identifying any individual. The majority of the bodies I examined during my involvement over the next few years showed evidence of gunshot trauma, but not always. The state of the bodies hampered the examinations. Sometimes they had been interred for years prior to discovery so were in an advanced stage of decomposition. Also, a body's condition depended to some extent on whether it was at the bottom of the grave or near the top: that affected the rate of decomposition, and whether or not we could identify a definite cause of death.

Normally I would begin a postmortem by examining the body from top to toe, noting its features and anything that might be useful in identification, as well as describing the clothing, then proceed to look for injuries, paying special attention to those that might have caused death. When dealing with the mass graves, the assumption was that these were unnatural deaths, but that had to be proven. The second assumption was that death was likely to have been due to gunshot trauma. But, of course, only when the postmortem is complete can the pathologist confirm or refute such allegations.

I approached these examinations exactly as I would in any potential murder. Once the preliminary examination is complete in a potential shooting I will examine the clothing for holes that indicate that the deceased has been struck by a bullet, then check the surface of the body for holes indicating the entry or exit of a bullet, X-ray the body to locate any bullet retained within it and finally open it to see the internal damage and find any retained bullet.

But the conditions here weren't normal. The clothing was badly damaged or missing, the bodies were badly decomposed, skin sloughing off, and there was often damage caused postmortem in the grave or when bodies were moved *en masse* to another burial site, a secondary grave. Also, the X-ray machine, a fluoroscope, wasn't working when I was there, hampering my ability to 'see' metal inside the bodies. I've performed postmortems in graveyards on exhumed bodies, in sheds, fields and an aircraft hangar so the issues in that makeshift mortuary weren't going to stop me doing my best.

Clothing was removed and examined in great detail, a full description was made, down to the number of buttons and the colour of thread used to sew them on, but also, if possible, whether there was any damage that could be related to an injury. We also checked for anything that might suggest blindfolds or restraints had been applied. The bodies ranged from grey putty-like unidentifiable humans to skeletalised remains, which hampered finding damage that might have been inflicted and responsible for death.

With no X-ray to identify bullets, I resorted to looking for bone damage that might have been due to a bullet and, as the internal organs were largely sludge, feeling around the soft tissues in that area for anything that might be a bullet. Sometimes I was lucky enough to see some green discoloration indicating a copper-coated bullet nearby. In some cases, particularly if there was head injury, the damage to bone was sufficiently typical of bullet trauma for me to be confident that death was due to a gunshot, even in the absence of a bullet. In many cases, though, there was insufficient evidence to give a definitive cause of death and I had to note it as 'Undetermined'. Not satisfactory but truthful.

Some of the investigators appointed by the UN to look into possible war crimes thought that was unhelpful and could be detrimental to their case, but my British colleagues and I felt that, even if you could only confirm that a percentage of the bodies from a mass grave had been fatally shot, the circumstances and the postmortem findings were more than sufficient to support that these were war crimes.

Over the next few years, having survived that trip, I continued to support the UN war-crimes work in former Yugoslavia. The facilities in Visoko and Zagreb were a vast improvement on Tuzla, with all mod cons, including electricity. The work was essentially the same, documenting everything, attempting to identify the deceased and determining how they had died. At any time there could be six or more pathologists of different nationalities working in the mortuary, as well as a dozen or so anthropologists. As time passed, the bodies were found to be in a worse condition, largely disintegrating and often reduced to bare bones, hence the huge number of anthropologists required to try to identify the remains, ageing, sexing and scouring for any clue as to who this might have been.

Despite the working conditions and an overwhelming sadness due to what we witnessed, we had a common cause: to identify the deceased in the hope of bringing justice to them and their families. We had descriptions, provided by the relatives, of those missing since the onset of the war, and the 'anthros' checked all our findings against them. Every so often we would have a potential identity. That was what it was about for me. Giving the body back to the family.

During our visits to Visoko we were living in the homes of local families. Usually only females and children were left in the home, the men missing, most presumed dead. The women appreciated what we were doing and wanted to take care of us. I stayed with the same family on my visits. I don't think it was because they were particularly fond of me – the language barrier meant we did no more than nod and smile at one another – but, being small and not fond of breakfast, I was probably the cheapest of all to keep, and I guess every penny counted for those women trying to carry on without their menfolk. But it suited both parties.

I don't know how many of the families ever got closure, but we tried. Since then DNA analyses have been ongoing on the samples taken at the postmortems, and thousands of the bodies from the mass graves have been identified.

DNA is now routinely used to identify bodies. Nowadays it is fast and efficient and, importantly, conclusive, but not always possible, unfortunately, when we need it most. There are still issues with some decomposed or skeletonised remains and fire fatalities. When I became a forensic pathologist in 1985, DNA was not part of our toolkit for identifying bodies. It was first used in a criminal case in the late 1980s in the USA. Everyone was very excited by the new technology that would revolutionise criminal investigations. But there were sceptics, me included. The forensic science laboratory required copious amounts of blood and tissue to produce a profile, and to what end? In the early days, it wasn't much help in the investigation of homicides, but within a couple of years we were beginning to appreciate its use in other cases, particularly rapes and sex-related homicides.

In the majority of cases the DNA profile generated is from the genetic material in the nucleus of cells. Half of this material is passed from the mother and half from the father, which means that an unknown person can be identified by comparing their profile with their parents, siblings or children. Nuclear DNA is sometimes not present in sufficient quantities to generate a full profile. There may be a difficulty when bodies are severely burned in fires or in old or skeletal remains when nuclear DNA cannot be extracted from the tissues. In those cases the option is to extract mitochondrial DNA. This is genetic material passed down from the mother in the cellular material that surrounds the nucleus of the egg; sperm is a nucleus without other cellular material.

Mitochondria are organelles within the cell and they are abundant and therefore an option when nuclear material is scarce. They are present in hair, bones and teeth, all that remains in some cases. This will identify you as part of a maternal tribe. Your mother and her siblings, you and your siblings share the same mitochondrial DNA. It is not unique to you in the same way as your nuclear DNA identifies you and you alone, but that level of discrimination is sufficient in most instances, particularly when identifying a single body. Similarly, Y-chromosome DNA is passed from father to son and may be useful, in the absence of a full nuclear DNA profile, to identify an unknown male.

It's not my area of expertise, and while I understand the science behind this, I still don't comprehend how the percentages of certainty are arrived at. At least I understand blood grouping and how their numbers are worked out. There are eight blood groups, the most common being O+, which includes just under 40 per cent of the UK population and just under 50 per cent of the Irish population. The next highest is A+, and so on. The majority of us are rhesus positive, about 85 per cent. Prior to DNA evidence, these figures were accepted by the courts as positively identifying someone; of course, it was more certain if you were one of the 15 per cent of the population who are rhesus negative. Blood grouping is a little more complex than that and there are various subgroups, but in the old days finding that someone had a particular blood group was accepted by the courts as sufficient to identify them or conclusively link them to a crime. In hindsight this was a woeful standard of proof.

Nowadays, DNA has considerably improved our level of certainty in identifying an individual. Despite that, forensic scientists are careful with the language they use when giving evidence in court; they never positively identify a particular individual, but express that the chance of this particular DNA profile belonging to another individual is slim to none, or words to that effect.

The techniques used to provide a DNA profile were refined over time and now, potentially, a profile can be generated from a single cell. In reality, forensic investigations are at a stage where it is possible that a DNA profile can be generated from the few cells transferred from merely touching a person, no need for the transfer of bodily fluids such as semen or blood.

This means we have to think carefully before we even approach a body at the scene. What is important in this death? Identification of the deceased? Cause of death? Forensic evidence, which could identify the killer? We need to discuss our forensic strategy before there is any potential that we could contaminate the evidence. Is this a sex-related homicide? If so, there may be semen or other body fluids on the body, which will be picked up by our standard samples and swabs. But in this type of case the deceased might have been manually strangled and therefore there is potential to gain DNA evidence from the neck. In other cases if the body appears to have been moved after death, often in an attempt to conceal it, the wrists or ankles could have been grabbed to pull it. Similarly the investigating team, myself included, take great pains not to deposit our DNA on the body, hence the coveralls and masks. DNA profiling has greatly improved in efficiency and availability and we are grateful for the endeavours of the forensic science laboratories that have made it possible to identify bodies within a day or so.

In Dublin in 1981, on Valentine's night, there was a fire in the Stardust nightclub. Forty-eight young people died. There have been multiple inquiries into the events of that night by the gardaí, the coroner, and by and on behalf of the families, but it is not for me to determine why the fire broke out or what went wrong that so many perished. This happened long before I moved to Ireland so I know only what has been reported in the media. Had I been living in Dublin I might have been there that night as it was my twenty-sixth birthday.

Postmortems were carried out on the victims but unfortunately, due to the ferocity of the fire, five of the bodies were deemed unidentifiable. DNA was not an option in those days and there was no forensic anthropologist. There was a forensic dentist, who charted the teeth of the victims, and the pathologists documented what could be useful for identification purposes, but despite that, the coroner was of the opinion that there was insufficient evidence to identify the five. The decision was made to bury them side by side, identified as the group of five individuals not identified. People like to know where their family member is buried. Many find it comforting to visit the grave, and it is not good enough to point out a general area and say that their family member is there somewhere. The families in this case campaigned tirelessly for an independent investigation into the fire and for the five unidentified to be formally identified.

In 2007 Brian Farrell, the Dublin coroner, agreed to the exhumation of the five unidentified victims of the Stardust fire and asked me, as state pathologist, and Laureen Buckley, the forensic anthropologist, to assist. We weren't 100 per cent sure that the remains could be identified from DNA, but we thought there might be other identifying features that would help. We could not make any promises as we had no idea what state the remains were in, given they had been so badly damaged by the fire to be considered unidentifiable, had been subject to a postmortem dissection and had been interred for around twenty-five years. But I always think you have to try.

We carefully exhumed the coffins and removed them to Dublin City Mortuary for examination.

Although the coffins were in a poor state, the bodies were still contained within them. Laureen and I worked in tandem, and despite our initial concerns and the passage of time, we managed to get a fair amount of information. By the end of our physical examination of the remains we had a good idea of the identity of each body. Science had moved on since 1981 and confirmation might be possible. DNA analysis was available to us and the families were more than willing to provide samples for comparison.

We sent bone samples from the remains to a specialist laboratory and, as we had suspected, the analyses were not straightforward: the laboratory could not extract nuclear DNA, but succeeded in isolating mitochondrial DNA. If the unidentified persons in the Stardust fire had been closely related, mitochondrial DNA would have only identified the bodies as being from the same maternal line, so siblings and cousins could not have been separated from one another on that basis alone. Other identifying features would have had to be taken into consideration. In this instance, the mitochondrial DNA analyses, with other information from the postmortems, was sufficient to identify each body. At long last the relatives had their own grave to visit.

The relative non-specificity of maternal DNA might have been an issue in identifying the victims of a fire in a halting site in Carrickmines in 2015. Five adults and five children perished, and one of the women was pregnant. A monumental tragedy. As with the Stardust fire, the effects of the blaze on the bodies were devastating, not only precluding visual identification of the individuals but also hampering DNA analysis. We knew from the start that the potential problem would be positive identification of the children, particularly two young brothers who were close in age, if we had to rely on mitochondrial DNA analysis. Maternal DNA alone would not indicate which child was which.

Three forensic pathologists, Margot Bolster, Linda Mullen and I, forensic anthropologist Laureen Buckley, and forensic dentist Mary Clarke were involved in the postmortems, the aim being to get as much information as we could to identify each body accurately.

The gardaí, in particular the Technical Bureau, were also heavily involved: the coroner had categorised the fire as a major incident. Each body was scrutinised: shape and colour of eyes, shape of nose, position and shape of ears, height, weight, burned remnants of clothing, moles, scars, any hint of previous accidents or illnesses, and crucially a dental examination. The pattern of eruption of baby teeth in the two young boys made it possible to confirm their identities without any doubt. The identification of the others was straightforward, using the information from the scene and the postmortem findings, and was confirmed by DNA.

Some cases prove a real challenge in regard to identification of the deceased, those where there is little left but bones or where only part of a body is recovered, and we may resort to other scientific means. The most common is radiology, the forensic pathologist's friend since 1895 when Wilhelm Roentgen discovered X-rays. While doctors were reticent about using this new technology in treatment, X-rays were being used within a year in criminal cases. Now we can use X-rays of the teeth and skull to help identify someone, or of the hips, for example, to detect metal prostheses.

Every year bodies are found that are not identified and no one comes forward to claim them. There is always the hope that eventually someone will look for them, but in the meantime the coroner will arrange for the body to be buried, the grave awaiting a nameplate. He or she will try by all means to identify the deceased but it may be impossible. Or not. Sometimes it takes just one person willing to go the extra mile and not give up.

In 2010 a human skull was brought ashore in Wexford by a fishing trawler. Body parts, human or animal, are not uncommonly caught in fishing nets. Generally, if human, it is likely someone who has gone overboard from a fishing boat or other vessel. Usually a knowledge of the waterways, tides and flow can help pinpoint where the person may have come from. It can also predict where a body is likely to be washed up if the point of entry is known, whether an accidental or deliberate drowning.

Initially there was nothing to suggest that this was anything other than the skull of some unfortunate man lost at sea, so it was not treated as suspicious but as an exercise in identification. With that in mind Laureen Buckley was asked to make a preliminary examination to see if she could help with identification.

What the garda did not expect was that while Laureen could identify the skull as possibly that of a middle-aged female, she was concerned that it was fractured, with a large crack on one side. At this point the death was deemed suspicious. As state pathologist I was asked to come down and have a look. I had to agree with Laureen on both counts, the skull was female and damaged. It was almost devoid of tissue and still had the upper two cervical vertebrae attached. The tissue remaining showed the soapy, waxy change that indicated it had been in the water for weeks, months or years. There was a 17.5cm crack fracture on the right side, above the 'ear', and internally there was dark staining of the dura, the thick tissue lining the skull, likely bloodstaining. There was also a crack in the roof of the right eye socket. This had the hallmarks of a perimortem fracture, occurring at or around the time of her death. Many of the woman's teeth were still present and there was a crown on her upper left sixth tooth. I couldn't tell whether the crack fracture at the side had occurred before she went into the water, on the way in or once she was in the water, possibly struck by a boat. So, her death might have been accidental but I couldn't exclude the possibility that she had been struck on the head and either incapacitated or fatally injured and was then dumped in the sea. Or she might have gone in of her own accord. The key was to find out who she was and then how she had come to be in the water off the coast of Ireland.

The state of the skull suggested she had been in the water for months at least. The first port of call in these circumstances is to check for missing persons in Ireland over the last few years. No woman from anywhere in Ireland who had been reported missing matched. For many, that would have been the end of the road, investigation closed, but not for Detective Garda Gerry Kealy, an intrepid investigator who made it his mission to pursue the identification of all unidentified remains in his region to a satisfactory conclusion, if possible. Now that it seemed unlikely this woman was local he had to widen his search. To do so, he had to get as much information as he could about her from her skull, which meant accessing other methods of investigation that were not mainstream and sometimes very expensive.

First stage, get a better timeline: when did this person die? One method of determining how long someone has been dead is by measuring the levels of radioactive isotopes in the tissues. The isotopes most commonly examined in forensic cases are those of carbon and strontium. A laboratory in Northern Ireland carries out carbon dating and strontium analyses; the results are used to determine when a person lived. Carbon dating is used for archaeological specimens from as far back as about sixty thousand years, but it is not accurate when dealing with more recent remains.

The cut-off point for the forensic investigation of a death is up to seventy years, although this varies and some countries have no great interest after forty years. Perhaps in the UK and Ireland we are a little more optimistic as regards our lifespan, but we have to be realistic: if a person died more than fifty years ago, and appears to have been murdered, what are the chances of the perpetrator still being alive? We have to be pragmatic. Would a costly investigation, with a negligible chance of success, be justified? Not a decision I have to make, but I will still carry out a detailed examination: the family deserve to know what happened to their relative, even if that person died a long time ago.

The results of the isotope analyses confirmed that this was a modern skull, recent, its owner probably dead only a few years. That was important: if this was a suspicious death her family and any potential assailant were likely to be alive. Facial reconstruction can be helpful when trying to identify human remains. An ex-colleague of mine, Dame Sue Black, was then head of the world-renowned forensic anthropology unit in Dundee, which included experts in facial reconstruction. I'd seen the results in other cases: pretty impressive. Gerry arranged for this to be done.

Meanwhile, I had cut out a small piece of bone and sent this, with a tooth, for DNA analysis, hoping that at some point the family would be found and we would be able to confirm her identity by comparing the DNA analysis from the skull with that of putative relatives.

Gerry had also heard of a chap who would do a stable isotope analysis of a tooth, which could determine the person's diet and therefore where they had been living. The results of determining the ratio of stable isotopes to normal atoms of oxygen, carbon and nitrogen in the enamel of the second molar can be used to determine the diet and potential source of water drunk during the formative years of the tooth's development, that is from seven to sixteen years old. Each region shows specific ratios, and by using all three elements, it was hoped to narrow down the area where she had lived as a child and teenager. The expert's analysis pointed to the deceased having lived in North America. But the search there proved futile, for reasons that only became apparent once the woman was identified.

Meanwhile, dental examination confirmed she had been over forty, and another anthropologist, René Gapert, had helped to confirm that she was Caucasian and also discovered a few reddish brown hairs embedded in an eye socket. Radiology showed arthritis of her neck and a peculiarity likely to cause fainting. A 'picture' of this woman was beginning to emerge, which was transcribed onto the page when facial reconstruction was complete.

Gerry continued his quest, approaching hundreds of doctors and dentists in the area. He sent all the information he had to Interpol to widen the search in Europe. The breakthrough came with a search of the UK database of women reported missing there over the last few years. One potential match was a middle-aged female with a history of depression who had been reported missing by her husband a year or so earlier, four months before the skull was caught in the trawler's net. Her car had been found close to the cliffs in Wales and it was assumed she had gone into the sea. Local searches had been unsuccessful, no body was recovered, and she was recorded as missing, presumed drowned.

Could this be our woman? Was it possible that she could have ended up so close to Ireland? There was nothing in her description that did not fit with the skull from the trawler. A photograph of her was not an identical match with the model produced in the Dundee Laboratory, although there were some similarities. However, she had never lived in the USA. DNA comparison of a profile from the skull and a profile obtained from the missing woman's glasses clinched it – it was a positive match.

It transpired that this woman had suffered from Addison's disease, one side-effect being that it affects the metabolism of nutrients and therefore may have skewed the results of the isotope analysis. This condition is treated with steroids, which may cause the patient to develop a 'moon face' that could not have been predicted by those carrying out facial reconstruction. Such investigations are an adjunct to identification, not the answer. All science has limitations.

Although the rest of her body was unlikely to be found, it was reasonable to assume she had fallen from the cliff edge into the sea and the fracture of the skull was due to her head striking the rocks below the cliff. Mercifully her death would have been rapid. Sad to think she had taken her own life but her husband was relieved to have her death confirmed and to have her, or at least part of her, to bury.

This was another mystery solved. There is never a happy ending in these circumstances, but at least a name had been restored to its rightful owner and the deceased returned to her family.

5

Mortuary

THE MAJORITY OF DEATHS ARE due to natural causes. Unfortunately, in some instances, even when death is almost certainly due to a heart attack or some chronic disease and the deceased was in their eighties, the coroner will request a postmortem examination, usually because the subject hadn't seen a doctor for over a month. Therefore, before a postmortem is carried out the pathologist usually has a good idea of what to expect, but sometimes things are not as they had seemed.

On this occasion a young man was brought into the mortuary from home. He lived alone, had a history of drug-taking and alcohol abuse. A friend had found him dead seated in an armchair. He was covered with blood, always a cause for concern. The gardaí first on the scene called in a doctor to pronounce death: he was told about the man's background, examined the body and found no injuries to his chest, abdomen or scalp that might have accounted for the blood coating his face, hands and clothes. He made a tentative diagnosis of massive gastrointestinal haemorrhage, alcohol-related, a bleeding ulcer or ruptured varices, the dilated veins in the oesophagus a complication of cirrhosis of the liver. At any rate no one had any real concern regarding the circumstances of the death. The coroner requested a postmortem to confirm the cause.

Within a few minutes of starting the postmortem, I became very concerned as to the circumstances of this man's death. As I scrubbed the congealed blood from his face and hands its source became apparent. In the centre of his forehead there was a gaping hole of about a centimetre across. I immediately telephoned the coroner and the local detective superintendent to inform them that what had been treated as a natural death was in fact suspicious. My scalpel went down and I waited for the Technical Bureau to arrive before I could continue.

Apart from a few minor and inconsequential bruises on his legs the only finding was the laceration on the forehead. There was no fracture of the skull and no bleeding inside the skull or trauma to the brain. Despite his history of drug and alcohol abuse, he had been relatively healthy with no evidence of liver disease or other alcohol-related gut problems. His death was simply due to haemorrhaging from the wound. The doctor was doubtful of my findings so I invited him to come and see the wound for himself. He declined. Whether I was right or wrong, nothing would entice him into the mortuary. A murder inquiry was set in motion; the system had worked.

A few days later a man handed himself in admitting he had thumped a man and knocked him out but the ring he had been wearing at the time had burst the skin on his forehead. His conscience was pricking him.

In general, mortuaries are tucked away at the backs of hospitals, perhaps to avoid either upsetting patients or acknowledging that some patients do not leave by the front door. If you ever have to seek one out, go to the back of the oldest building on site and look for the boiler house. The mortuary will be next to it. It's always the last department to get funding but why should the dead be short-changed? Instead of skulking around dark corridors when a loved one dies, there should be a modern, bright, clean and welcoming area to which families and friends are directed, in an effort to make them more comfortable at a trying time and reassure them that the deceased is being treated with the respect they deserve. Most hospitals now have facilities that would rival a sterile operating theatre but some mortuaries still fall a little short.

Once the body enters the mortuary the pathologist takes charge of the situation. It is always a team collaboration but the pathologist is hands-on. I have to ensure that all relevant forensic evidence is collected, every stray hair or fibre, any debris attached or any smear of blood or fluid, body or otherwise, on the clothes or the body. I scrutinise its surface for any tiny mark or injury before I explore inside. I could not practise without assistance in the mortuary from an anatomical pathology technician (APT). In the early days they were known as 'slab men', and usually had another role in the hospital, in the laboratories or as a porter, and volunteered to assist in the mortuary, basically cleaning up after the pathologist. There was no training and certainly no thanks. When I started in pathology, training for technicians had been introduced in hospital mortuaries, and over the last twenty years their role has been recognised.

When I started in the city mortuary in Glasgow, Jackie, Fenton and Alex had no formal qualifications but over the next few years I encouraged the new recruits, Brian and Sandie, to study. It's a difficult job, not for the faint-hearted, and APTs deserve recognition for everything they do, not just in the mortuary but with relatives at the most vulnerable time in their lives. I cannot thank them enough. Apart from their assistance during postmortems, there were little acts of kindness, such as building a platform for me to stand on so I could reach the mortuary table comfortably, filling buckets of hot water for me to stand in when it was freezing in winter and there was no heating in the mortuary, and don't forget the tea and cakes. I missed them more than the pathologists when I left for Ireland. Luckily for me, the APTs in Ireland were just as welcoming and accommodating.

In the early years most of my work was in Dublin, and Carl Lyon, the APT in Dublin City Mortuary, became my right-hand person, swiftly followed by Tricia Graham; we became a tight little team. Outside Dublin, John in Limerick and Dan and his boys in Cork, in particular, were excellent mortuary mates. Slab men no longer, they are all highly trained and made my life so much easier.

It wasn't only the expertise of the APTs that was unappreciated by hospitals and medical practitioners: the role of the pathologist was not recognised. Historically, any doctor, commonly general practitioners and surgeons, could be instructed to carry out postmortems, even though they had had no specific training. Slowly they were replaced by trained pathologists and it was in the 1970s in the UK that it was decided only doctors with special training in forensic pathology should be involved in the investigation of homicides. In England and Wales they were called Home Office pathologists. In Scotland the scope was widened to include any natural or unnatural death being investigated by the procurator fiscal, and four centres were set up in Edinburgh, Glasgow, Aberdeen and Dundee. Around this time changes were also afoot in Ireland and it was not long until Jack Harbison was appointed state pathologist. Thus began the era of modern forensic pathology in the UK and Ireland.

At the early stage in an investigation of a death, there is usually little information as to the circumstances surrounding it, and what information there is still has to be verified. I usually prefer to ignore what is no more than speculation and let the body speak for itself. As always, I strive to be independent and unbiased. Often difficult when the crowd in the mortuary butt in with their own theories. It may be days, weeks or even months before I realise the relevance of the smallest of injuries on a body. In fact, it is often the insignificant injuries that reveal most about the actual circumstances of a death. The tiny fingertip bruise on the inside of the upper arm caused by it being grabbed, the small scratch on the neck, perhaps from a fingernail. Each injury tells a story but, to get the big picture, all the injuries have to be taken into consideration in a search for patterns that will reveal what happened on the fateful day or night. In most cases the cause of death is not in dispute: the man in the street could identify that someone was shot, stabbed or brutally beaten. But that's the easy part. The more difficult part is marrying the fatal injury with the others present, the findings at the scene and any reliable information about the death. It's the pathologist's job to help paint that big picture, to be able to play out the scenario, blow by blow, shot by shot, stab by stab.

Many bodies are brought to my attention not because they have obviously been murdered but because there is something of concern. It may be that the deceased or their family had been brought to the attention of the police or social services in the past; an allegation of a recent minor assault; their state of dress or undress; an injury or injuries. Such deaths are described as 'suspicious'. In Ireland there are around thirty thousand deaths every year, most from natural causes such as heart and related vascular diseases and cancers. About half of all deaths are reported to the coroner but only about a third to a half of those will be investigated by the coroner and a postmortem examination carried out.

In the majority of cases, the postmortem will confirm that the death was due to natural causes and no further action is required. The remaining two thousand or so represent accidental deaths, suicides, deaths in hospital, drug-related deaths, deaths at work and so on, but only a small proportion of these, around two hundred each year, are identified as suspicious, or possible homicides. In reality the homicide rate remains fairly stable at between fifty and seventy per year in Ireland.

The basic postmortem always includes a full external examination, documenting the person's features, as well as all marks or injuries and evidence of natural disease. Only then will the internal organs be examined, from the brain to the bladder and everything in between. Of course, the older the person was at death, the more likely there will be wear and tear of the organs. Sometimes it is not so much 'What did they die of?' but 'How did they keep going for so long?'

The postmortem is a snapshot of the last moment of life. It tells you the state of the organs at the time of death. Like looking at a photograph taken on a night out showing happy faces, but not the events leading up to it or what happened next: the best friends arguing about whose turn it was to pay for the taxi, the boyfriend about to proposition his girlfriend's friend, the guy who got into an argument and ended up in A&E. I cannot tell if the person had been complaining of pain, had been failing over the past week, would have survived if they had sought medical treatment sooner. I can tell you what pathology was present at the time of the person's death and what could have given rise to it. Most importantly, whether or not it could have caused the person's death.

If someone has had heart disease for years, what was so different about the day of their death that caused the heart to fail at that particular time? An example is the stress-associated heart attack. Every year there will be one or two instances where an older person is involved in a stressful incident that causes them to collapse and die. It might be a heated argument, a bag-snatch or a minor scuffle. Nothing that would be expected to have a fatal outcome. All of those deaths have in common postmortem evidence of significant heart disease, even if it had not been diagnosed during their life. Due to that gloopy porridge-like material, atheroma, and possibly a 'touch' of high blood pressure, the blood supply to the heart muscle has become compromised. Under the person's normal conditions enough blood was getting through to keep them free of symptoms, but in a stressful situation the heart quickens and the blood pressure starts to rise, putting extra strain on the heart. The result is a heart attack, collapse and death. Adrenalin is mighty useful at giving us an extra boost when the chips are down, but sometimes it can be detrimental.

The diagnosis is easy to make due to the close

association between an incident and the sudden collapse of an individual. Well, it's easy for the pathologist but not for the law enforcers. Do they charge the other person involved in the fracas with causing a death, a homicide? The sad fact is that if the deceased had been running late and made a sprint for a bus the outcome might have been the same. Stress is stress.

Facing death on a daily basis must have some effect. I don't have nightmares about horrendously mangled bodies and zombies attacking me. When I lose sleep it's because I'm processing my postmortem findings and trying to make sense of them. I feel a tremendous responsibility to get things right, not only for the deceased person but also for their family. Pathology is no different from most professions in that 90 per cent of the work is straightforward: it is the other 10 per cent that presents the challenge. The majority of deaths are uncomplicated, but there are always cases where you have no answer.

Some pathological diagnoses are always unsatisfactory and relate mainly to the deaths of the most vulnerable in the population: babies and young persons. Accidental deaths, suicides and homicides must be very difficult to come to terms with, but I can try to explain to the family what happened to their nearest and dearest.

The worst diagnosis I can give to a family is that the cause of death is 'undetermined'. We can dress it up, using terms such as 'cot death' or 'sudden infant death syndrome' (SIDS), in babies, or 'sudden arrythmogenic disorder syndrome', SADS, in young men and women. Those diagnoses deliver a life sentence to that family. What about my other children? Will it happen again? Should I have more children? Whose fault was it? My faulty genes or yours?

Mercifully, researchers are dedicated to trying to get to the bottom of these deaths. New genetic mutations are being discovered, which take us closer to finding the cause of death in babies and young persons. Sometimes, as in the case of SIDS, the research identified risk factors other than faulty genes, faulty information given to new mums. Simple instructions on making sure the baby was not kept too warm or placed face down in the cot had a dramatic effect and the number of baby deaths dropped considerably. But the search continues.

In the majority of cases the cause of death is pretty straightforward: a stab wound to the chest, a gunshot wound to the head, a major blunt-instrument trauma. There are eye-witness accounts and forensic evidence identifying the perpetrator – slam dunk!

Sometimes, though, even such open and closed cases can throw up a few curve-balls. Eye-witnesses may not agree with one another. When things happen in an extremely short period of time people may not see everything and may believe they saw something that did not happen. The postmortem may reveal injuries that could not have been inflicted in the manner described.

A case in point was that of a young child struck by a vehicle. The child ran into the path of the vehicle and, even though it was not travelling at great speed, a collision could not be avoided. There were many witnesses and some described their horror at seeing the child catapulted into the air. The postmortem findings refuted those eye-witness accounts: the child was not lifted into the air on impact. He was knocked down and run over. Still, not something any of us would choose to witness.

In pedestrian road fatalities there is usually no doubt that death was due to a severe head injury, most commonly from impact with the ground, or crushing of the chest on being run over. But who was at fault? Driver versus pedestrian: not an even contest. Is the driver of the vehicle a reliable witness? 'He ran out in front of me', 'I was only doing thirty', 'I tried to avoid him/her' . . . This is where the science comes in. Experts on road-traffic collisions can analyse marks on the road and any debris from a vehicle and can determine where the impact took place, at what speed the vehicle was travelling, the braking distance and so on. The pathologist's examination will concentrate on the pattern of injuries: which part of the body the vehicle struck first and what happened to the body thereafter.

Typically, when an ordinary saloon car hits a pedestrian, the bumper will strike the legs, the exact point depending on the individual's height. And, again depending on their height and therefore their centre of gravity, they may be lifted up and propelled back over the vehicle or knocked over by the force of the impact. If lifted, they may collide with some part of the vehicle and/or the road. Each impact leaves tell-tale signs. Drawing from their experience the pathologist can offer an opinion on the dynamics of the incident. From what direction was the person crossing the road? Were they struck full on, thrown into the air or knocked down and run over? Collating the examinations of the scene, vehicle and deceased should give a fairly clear picture of what happened.

Does that match the eye-witness accounts or the version of events given by the driver? In one case the driver, and a couple of eye-witnesses, said that the deceased, a teenager, sprang off the pavement and sprinted across the road in front of the vehicle, which was slowing as the traffic lights ahead had turned red. The postmortem showed that both shin bones of the young man were fractured just above the ankle. Normally we walk by raising one leg up, planting it back down, repeat. If struck by a vehicle I expect the standing leg to be hit at about bumper height, around the knees in an adult. The raised leg, if struck, will show an injury at a lower level. The site of injury to the legs of the young man was below bumper level. He must have been running like a gazelle, both legs in the air, when he was struck, confirming the driver's account.

That's why we do postmortems, even when the cause of death is obvious to everyone involved in the investigation. It's looking for that little bit extra, the answer to the question no one has thought to ask . . . yet.

Detailing the injuries in murder cases is laborious. Surprisingly, shooting incidents are the cleanest, although not always the quickest. Bullets leave a small hole on the outside but as they travel through the body their energy has a devastating effect, ripping gaping tunnels through the organs. The shock wave produced can cause almost instant death even if the bullet doesn't go through the brain but is close enough, striking the face or neck, the ripples disrupting the brainstem and its vital centres. Shotguns are even more vicious when fired at close quarters, exploding the head or leaving fist-sized holes in the body and shredding the heart and lungs. With shooting incidents, the cause of death is not difficult. The challenge is imagining the sequence of events: how far away was the shooter? How many shots were fired? Was the victim sitting, standing, running away? And, of course, we want to recover the evidence: the bullets.

It sometimes isn't as easy as you would think to find a bullet inside the body. They can get trapped in bone, lost in a sea of blood and mangled tissue. The easiest way to identify a bullet, or any metal, in a body is to X-ray it, the only problem being that most mortuaries don't have such equipment. We have to rely on the hospital radiology departments to assist us, but they have far more pressing business: live patients. That's why we may be found skulking around the X-ray departments in the dead of night when the patients are tucked up in bed.

In all my years no radiology department has ever declined to X-ray a body. My thanks to them all, they have saved me a lot of blood, sweat and tears trying to locate bullets. But even with the assistance of radiology, it may not be plain sailing. I have been fooled by a stray or loose bullet, which, on a two-dimensional X-ray, appears to be in a precise location but is in fact lying under the body or caught in the folds of the clothing, and 'disappeared' when I went looking for it inside the body. Always check the body bag and the clothing.

Nowadays more sophisticated techniques are being used, and in Dublin the coroner has access to CT scanning and a dedicated team of radiographers and radiologists. This can greatly assist the pathologist in determining the tracks of the bullets into and through the body in order to determine their trajectory. In doing so it may be possible to build a picture of the shooting incident: random versus deliberate close-range shots, a targeted attack, an execution or even the wrong target. I've seen it all. The injuries may help point the police in the right direction.

In Scotland shootings were uncommon in the 1980s, but with the increasing drug trade, they became more common in the 1990s. Often tit for tat. Ireland is very different. Shotguns are prevalent in the farming community and easily available. The downside is that they are commonly used in suicide. In Glasgow shotguns are in short supply, rat poison being the method of choice for getting rid of vermin. Before I moved to Ireland I had seen relatively few shotgun fatalities.

Northern Ireland has a reputation for gun violence, which, as far as the UK was, and to some extent still is, concerned, meant the whole of Ireland. In Scotland, this was probably because most travelled to Ireland by ferry, landing in the ports around Belfast to be met by the British Army. I remember well my first holiday with girlfriends from school, looking out the window of the bus at the soldiers on the streets. It could have been Beirut for all my fifteen-year-old self knew. But how times have changed. In the south we are now seeing more shootings than in Northern Ireland and most big cities in the UK.

Unlike Ireland, where the numbers of shootings, stabbings and head injuries are roughly the same, the principal murder mode in Scotland is stabbing. Glasgow in particular has a long-held tradition of knife crime, earning it the tag 'No Mean City'. I remember giving a lecture in Limerick and inadvertently referring to it as 'Stab City', quoting what I had read in the press. This provoked a rather terse response from the local TD to the effect that, coming from Glasgow, I was in no position to be 'throwing stones at glass houses'. Fair point, well made.

I became rather an expert on stab wounds. Although most stab wounds are inflicted by steak knives or hunting knives, anything with a point can be driven into the body – pencils, pens, screwdrivers and swords. I've seen them all. It is amazing how much information can be gleaned from examining one: the position on the body, the direction of the internal wound track, the size and shape of an individual wound and the number of wounds, all tell a tale. The pattern of injuries will help me to determine the positions of the parties during an assault, how a knife was wielded, the configuration of a blade, how many knives were used, whether there was a struggle or the injured party was overcome, then repeatedly stabbed.

The information from the postmortem won't alter the fact that death was due to a stab wound, or wounds, but may assist the police in their investigation, and determining the circumstances of an assault: self-defence, an 'accident' or a deliberate and sustained assault? In other words, manslaughter or murder? Generally, the greater the number of stab wounds the greater the intent, but not all deaths due to multiple stab wounds are homicides: some may be self-inflicted, as unlikely as that may seem to most people.

While the violence people can inflict on one another never ceases to amaze me, the violence people can inflict on themselves is even more surprising. Most of us are lucky enough never to suffer from severe depression, the despair that drives someone towards taking their own life. Family members will ask, 'Why would they do this?' I can't answer that question. No one can.

For the family, the person's mood may sometimes seem improved prior to that final act, which is especially poignant. But not all people suffering from depression get to that point. No assumption can ever be made that a person suffering from depression killed themselves. Each and every death has to be fully investigated before a diagnosis of suicide can be made. A medical diagnosis of depression may cloud the issue, but all other possibilities must be aired, the final decision resting with the coroner after all evidence is heard.

A man was found dead in a pool of blood in a locked cabin in a submarine at sea. His throat had been cut. He had a history of depression and had been rather withdrawn over the previous few days. It was suicide, wasn't it? But there was no obvious weapon in the room. So, was it homicide? I was sceptical that a body found in a locked room in a submarine, which had been at sea, could be entertained as a potential homicide. This was not a case for Poirot, more for Houdini. Sure enough, the photographs showed a small cabin awash with blood, but I reserved judgement until I could examine the body.

The man had obviously been dead for some hours; he was coated with a thick layer of congealed blood; and there was an obvious gaping wound on his neck. The forensic textbooks describe how to tell the difference between self-inflicted and homicidal wounds by looking for tentative injuries. These are small, shallow cuts around a larger, sometimes fatal wound, classically seen on the wrists when someone attempts suicide. Similar wounds may be present on the neck but the distinction between suicide and homicide is more difficult to determine in reality.

During the clean-up process I discovered multiple incised wounds on the neck, indicating possible self-inflicted trauma, as well as the obvious fatal injury. To confirm whether this was suicide or homicide, I examined the body for any other knife wounds, particularly on the arms. Cuts across the front of the wrists lend weight to a suicide whereas cuts along the edge of the forearms could indicate a struggle with a third party, these wounds defensive in nature. As I scrubbed at the stubborn bloodstains on the man's arms, I found within the sticky clot fusing his fingers together a small blade from a modern razor. How much intent, and patience, must it have taken to do sufficient damage to cause death with such a tiny implement? A dismantled razor was found in the cabin. Suicide.

Another similar case a few years earlier, in January 1997, had a very different outcome. Marion Ross, a middle-aged woman, had been living alone in the family home since her parents died. According to her family, she had a history of depression and other mental health issues. She was found dead in the hallway. There was blood on and around the body. The house had been secure with no evidence of a break-in. She had last been seen alive in the local town that morning where she was shopping. The police called a local doctor to pronounce death. He saw the wounds on her neck, which he thought could have been self-inflicted. The police called me, just to be sure. I agreed that multiple stab wounds on the neck might be self-inflicted, but a more common site would be the chest, targeting the heart. A pair of scissors was still embedded in the woman's neck – it's not uncommon in suicides that the weapon is still in the body. But . . .

While I waited for the scientists to finish around the body, I looked in the kitchen. Her shopping from that morning was still on the table. It was likely the scissors in her neck had come from the kitchen. Generally when someone decides to commit suicide it appears to have been considered. Why stab yourself in the hallway? Why not the kitchen, living room or bedroom? Why choose scissors when you've a drawer full of knives?

At last I was called to the body. Yes, the scissors

were embedded in her neck. Yes, there were multiple stab wounds on her neck. But when I looked at her face I noticed stab wounds to her eyes.

I summoned the investigating officer and said I was sorry but this looked like a homicide. And it was. Solving it entailed a long and difficult investigation for the police. It would appear that this had been a robbery gone wrong. Through a process of elimination a young man, who had been one of the team of builders working on an extension to the house a couple of years earlier, was charged with the murder, based on fingerprint evidence. His fingerprint was found at the scene and the fingerprint of the victim was found on a biscuit tin containing a fair quantity of money at his home.

This case became infamous because of a challenge to the fingerprint evidence, which led to changes in how fingerprints are identified. One of the fingerprints found at the scene was identified as that of a detective. In those days it was not unheard of that people would enter a scene without protective clothing, including gloves. So, an odd rogue fingerprint was no big deal, except the detective maintained she had never been to the scene. The fingerprint expert was adamant that he had correctly identified the print and the police officer was equally adamant that it could not be hers.

The young man was charged with the murder and the case went to court. He maintained evidence had been planted in his home, implying a police officer had 'fitted him up'. The jury accepted the evidence linking him with the death of Marion Ross and he was found guilty of the murder.

Following the trial there was an inquiry into the fingerprint of the detective. She was suspended pending an inquiry, and was later sacked. She was left fighting for her reputation and her position in the police.

As part of her defence she had the fingerprint evidence from the murder case reviewed by a fingerprint expert from the USA. Pat Wertheim stated that the fingerprint was not hers and that the method used to identify it was flawed. Wow! That put all us scientists on a back foot. Unfortunately, it is a trap we can all fall into, assuming that something is scientifically proven and therefore a fact.

At her trial for perjury, the fingerprint evidence presented on her behalf was challenged by the prosecution. But Pat Wertheim demonstrated that the Scottish method of fingerprint identification was based on opinion rather than fact. The method used at that time was the points-based system I mentioned earlier, the certainty of match depending on the number of matching characteristics between two prints, the optimal being sixteen. While there were similarities between the detective's print and that found at the scene, much more importantly, there were several dissimilarities. The print was not hers.

The detective was acquitted and cleared of all allegations of misconduct. The Scottish experts would not accept they were wrong but eventually there was a change in the methodology and the system used in the rest of the UK and in the USA was adopted: fingerprints are now identified on the basis of the quality and uniqueness of the print rather than similarities. This opened the opportunity of appeal for the accused, and the doubt regarding the fingerprint evidence led to his sentence being overturned. At present no one stands accused of the murder. On one hand an injustice has been righted but, on the other, no justice for the murder victim.

6

What Happened

THE SCALPEL GOES DOWN. THE gown is discarded. The chatter stops. Heads turn expectantly, like fledglings in a nest waiting for a tasty treat. 'Well, Doc, what happened? Have we got a murder on our hands?'

The next words out of my mouth will determine what happens to this investigation. Will they rush off, relieved that a murder inquiry has been aborted – 'Thanks, Doc. Until the next time'? Or will there be a resigned collective sigh, as they settle back in their chairs, pens poised to take notes, their minds stepping up a gear in readiness to start a murder investigation?

Once the postmortem is over it is time to

debrief the police. The postmortem is not the end of the process for the pathologist, even when the cause of death seems clear. There may be other tests to carry out: toxicology, if drink or drugs may have been involved; histology, biochemistry or bacteriology, if natural disease may have played a part. All of these investigations take time – days, weeks or even months. But the police cannot hold fire. Action needs to be taken *now*. Decisions have to be made *now*.

The postmortem process is laborious and intense. For several hours I scrutinise and dissect a body, ensuring I get every piece of information I can. This 'patient' cannot prompt me by pointing to the bit that hurts or telling me what was done to them, but the marks and injuries on the body speak as loudly to me as a voice. Like translating French, or sign language, I have been trained to interpret it. And I may have to think carefully about what I have seen and recorded before I can be sure that I've 'listened' to the deceased and understood exactly what happened to them.

Forensic pathologists vary in how they transcribe their findings at postmortem. Television, in particular, loves the drama of the over-table microphone, the pathologist using a foot pedal to operate it while talking to the ceiling. Few of us would trust this technology: tricky to manoeuvre and a disaster if it fails. Most of us use a hand-held Dictaphone, some dictate during the course of the autopsy, but others, like me, take copious notes and plot every mark and injury on body diagrams as we work. The diagrams will augment the photographs taken by the police, under my direction, during every stage of the procedure and will be a permanent record of the autopsy findings.

The written notes are my evidence, my findings at the time of the examination. My writing is appalling, like that of most doctors: we are always in a hurry. I'm also trying not to touch the paper, which is in close proximity to the body and at risk of getting messy with anything but the point of my pen. It doesn't always work. The notes are my enduring record of my findings, and over the following weeks I will hone them into a report, which will be sent to the coroner, the official postmortem report. I take it to court and read it to the judge and jury.

The information I give to the police at the time of the autopsy may just be dotting the *i*s or crossing the *t*s. From the first call, everyone knew we were dealing with a murder. On the other hand, I may be reassuring the police that this is not a murder, and proceed to explain the most likely sequence of events leading up to the death: accident, suicide or unusual natural death. Of course, it takes a long time to gain sufficient experience to be able to make such decisions: the more cases the pathologist deals with, the wider their experience, and the more confident they will become in making the decision, murder or not. I have always said that in a busy forensic department, where pathologists deal with all types of unnatural and sudden deaths, it probably will take about two years for them to have come across a wide enough spectrum not to be fazed by whatever comes through the doors.

But that is only the start of the training for a forensic pathologist. This is not the time to become complacent: it's the danger period. Some think that at this stage they know it all. No, no, no: now you have to prove yourself and be tested. A couple of tricky times in court at the hands of a wily defence barrister will soon knock the cockiness out of the 'young pretender', the fresh-faced forensic pathologist who thinks they have it sussed. Over the years most forensic pathologists realise that little in life is black and white, and so it is with death. Definite becomes probable, probable becomes possible, and possible becomes maybe or maybe not. And that is the reality of being a forensic pathologist.

Determining whether or not a death is a murder in the early stages of an investigation is probably the forensic pathologist's most valuable contribution. Murder investigations are hugely expensive: if such an investigation is unnecessary that expense can be curtailed, which is to everyone's benefit. That's also why a forensic pathologist must be available 24/7 and that we respond swiftly. Much as I have always hated being on call, I never hesitated when I was summoned and got there as soon as was humanly possible. I could never relax if I was on call, but as soon as one came it was game on.

Just as with the Scottish criminal-court verdicts, there is a third category of case: 'I'm not 100 per cent sure'. These cases will probably not turn out to have been a murder, but there is still some work to be done before we can all relax. This may be a simple blood test, a closer look down the microscope at some of the tissues, or consultation with another expert. But it might be as simple as considering the myriad of ways injuries could have been caused and whether they might have been accidental, self-inflicted or had to have been inflicted by a third party. Accident, suicide or murder.

I have always been a bit apologetic about making a living out of stating the obvious, but few want to do it. First, it is a case of describing the injuries, of which there are five basic forms. Bruises, grazes, lacerations are the blunt-force injuries due to the application of mechanical force, such as a blow to the body or the body impacting with the ground. The commonest weapons are fists and feet, which can do as much damage as some manufactured weapons. Cuts and stab wounds are the sharp injuries caused by something with a sharp edge or tip, the most obvious being a knife but penetrating injuries can be caused by any long, narrow object pushed forcefully into the body.

Then there are the more complex injuries, caused by gunshot and burning, or the combination injuries, a mix of blunt and sharp trauma, such as glass and axe injuries. And, of course, there will often be a mix of blunt, sharp and complex injuries in any homicide case.

The key to interpreting the injuries is the pattern of trauma: the type of injury, where the individual injuries are on the body and in relation to each other, then determining which, if any, was likely to have been fatal. If it had been, would it have caused immediate or rapid death or would the victim have been expected to survive for some time after the injury was inflicted? These facts will enable the pathologist to interpret the manner and circumstances of infliction of the injuries: accident, suicide or homicide.

When determining the cause of death the pathologist must consider the totality of the injuries and decide how they killed the victim. Was only one injury responsible? A premise favoured by the defence counsel: 'So, Doctor, the stab wound to the chest was the only fatal injury and the other [fifty] injuries [stab wounds] were incidental.' Or was death due to the combined effects of all the injuries? In certain circumstances one specific injury can be identified as the killer but, more often than not, many of the injuries sustained would have contributed to the death. To make that distinction the pathologist must decide on the mechanism of death in the circumstances.

Death is most commonly due to haemorrhage or injury to a vital organ. In some instances, particularly nowadays with rapid-response teams and trained paramedics capable of urgent emergency treatment at the scene, death is not inevitable, even with a stab wound to the heart, and the victim may make a full recovery. In recent years forensic pathologists have seen a reduction in cases with a single injury, particularly a stab wound, due to the improvement in medical services.

The cases arriving in the mortuary are more complex and more violent than before. Early resuscitation is not a guarantee of survival. Loss of blood sets off a chain of events in the body that cannot be resolved by blood transfusion alone. Litres and litres of blood are pumped into injured individuals in the hope that that will sustain them for long enough to allow the medical staff to correct the complications arising. The injuries continue bleeding until treated, which might necessitate internal surgery, but meantime loss of blood has caused the body temperature to drop, hypothermia. The body tries to rectify the situation, plugging holes in damaged vessels, the kidneys struggling to deal with the changes in the pH of the blood, but rapidly runs out of the necessary materials to do so, particularly platelets and clotting factors.

At this stage blood is pouring out as fast as it is being poured in – even the clots formed come under attack. The heart begins to flag and, even in young, previously healthy individuals, gives up. In some cases, there may be attempts to perform cardiac massage, which means opening the chest cavity. Medical staff don't give up on anyone without a fight, but at this stage death is inevitable. The trace fades. R.I.P.

Even when the medical staff successfully resuscitate the injured, they are not out of the woods. The body has been under immense strain. The most vulnerable organs are the brain, heart and kidneys: the extent of damage to them may not be immediately obvious and they may not fully recover. Brain injury, cardiac scarring and renal failure may result.

Other potential complications are pulmonary thromboembolism, a threat to anyone confined to bed, particularly if a lower limb injury requires immobilisation. Prophylaxis for prevention of deep-vein thrombosis, which causes pain and swelling of the leg, is now routinely given. As a result, the incidence of death due to the thrombus from the leg veins breaking off and circulating into the heart and lungs has been dramatically reduced. But after my failure to diagnose a pulmonary embolism at my first postmortem, I always check, just in case.

However, another form of embolism, foreign material in the circulation that blocks vessels, cannot be predicted or prevented. Fat embolism syndrome is a well-recognised complication of trauma, particularly fractures of the long bones, but also when there is extensive soft-tissue injury and even in victims of severe burns. The marrow from the broken bone or fat from pulverised fatty tissue may get into the torn blood vessels in the injured area, then into the general circulation and the pulmonary circulation. These little globules of fat may block the small vessels in the brain, the lungs, the kidneys and the skin. This happens to many trauma patients but usually the effects are trivial. Unfortunately, in a few people, within hours or perhaps up to two or three days later, there is a massive influx of fat globules into the circulation and they take a turn for the worse. They may become confused or breathless, and develop a distinctive haemorrhagic rash. The diagnosis can be made quickly via a urine sample. This will show tiny globules of fat in the urine. The only treatment is supportive, but the brain lesions and the lung damage may cause death.

An elderly man was brought into hospital after an ambulance was called. His son said he had found him collapsed on the floor. He complained that he had a sore arm and chest. X-rays confirmed he had a fracture of his left humerus. This did not require anything more than a sling.

More worrying was his chest. In the centre, over the breast bone there was a long, wide injury. An X-ray showed a fracture of the sternum. This could not be treated and he was kept in overnight for observation. The medical staff informed the police that they were concerned that, while his fractured arm might have occurred in a fall, the chest injury was unusual and he might have been assaulted.

Once he was up in the ward the police asked him a few questions about the circumstances. He admitted that he had had a row with his son in their kitchen. A chair was broken and the son struck his father with one of its legs. The elderly man said he did not want to press charges. The police asked if he would mind a police photographer taking photographs of his injuries. He agreed, and the photographs showed him sitting up in bed, smiling for the camera, his arm in a sling, his pyjama top open to reveal a large purple bruise covering the centre of his chest.

Twenty-four hours later he lay on the mortuary

table. Overnight his condition had deteriorated. He had become extremely breathless. He was given oxygen. It was assumed he had had a heart attack, not surprising given that his son had beaten him up. He did not respond and died quickly.

The police were concerned. An elderly man had died within a couple of days of being beaten up by his son. His wishes would no longer restrict their actions. I was asked to carry out a postmortem to determine the cause of death. Had he had a heart attack? Or was his death directly due to his injuries?

The postmortem confirmed the extent of the injuries as detailed by the doctors who had been treating him – no surprises there. He also had some narrowing of his coronary arteries but no scarring of the myocardium: the degree of heart disease was no more than would be expected in someone of his age. An unexpected finding was multiple small haemorrhages in the lungs and the brain. Could this be a case of fat embolism? The importance of such a diagnosis is that fat embolism is a direct complication of the injuries sustained. Whoever had inflicted the injuries had caused the death: a clear-cut diagnosis, which made the decision to charge the perpetrator with murder straightforward. In contrast, if death was due to pre-existing heart disease the connection between the assault and death would become more tenuous as the time between incident and death lengthened: to be certain of a charge of murder, there has to be a close temporal association.

To confirm the diagnosis of death caused by fat embolism syndrome, I took samples of the brain, lungs and kidneys to be examined under the microscope. The normal tissue processing for histological examination includes subjecting the tissue to chemicals, which would dissolve fat. However, as I had this diagnosis in mind, I asked my technician, Kate Clapperton, who ran a very efficient histology laboratory, to freeze pieces of fresh tissue and stain the sections with a dye that would show fat globules. Kate produced the slides within the day. The police were informed that the diagnosis had been confirmed. The son was charged with the murder of his father. He pleaded guilty to manslaughter on the day of the trial. He received a sentence commensurate with the enormity of his crime. I've never forgotten the photograph of that old man, smiling into the camera. I hope his son felt some remorse for his actions.

The cause of death is the major concern, at first,

but the next consideration is more important to the investigation of the death. Is it a homicide, or could there be some other explanation? The first chance to make the right call was at the scene. This is the second chance. Make a wrong decision and either a homicide is missed, and the perpetrator gets away scot-free, or a death is mistakenly classified as a homicide, and some poor person is unfairly accused. To hell with the expense of an unnecessary murder investigation, more worrying is a miscarriage of justice so forensic pathologists do not take this decision lightly. The decision as to whether or not this is or could be a homicide is made not only on the basis of the findings at postmortem but by taking into consideration the scene and all the information acquired by the investigating officers up to that point.

When preparing my report for court I always include the caveat 'should further information come to light, I may have to revise my opinion'. If the pathologist decides that this is not a homicide, the investigation into the death should not be aborted, but must continue until there is a satisfactory conclusion. There may be a scaling-back of police personnel and less urgency but there are still questions to be answered and the police must be able to reassure the family that there was a full inquiry, no evidence of third-party involvement, and that this was supported by the pathologist's findings. Most families are satisfied by this, but not all. Over the years I have seen a change in people's attitudes.

We have entered the era of a 'blame culture' in which no one takes responsibility for their actions, and when it comes to death someone, not the deceased, must be to blame. In some instances, families will have their own theories and are extremely unhappy if the police and I do not agree. They are frustrated by what they perceive is a lack of interest in the truth, and I am equally frustrated that they could believe I would try to cover up a homicide. Why would I? What is the advantage to me? None at all. Despite that, I will answer a family's queries and try to explain how and why I came to the decision I did. But sometimes it is still not enough and families spend years campaigning for cases to be reopened. No one rests in peace. In contrast, I am awed by the strength of those families who use their tragedy to influence changes that will benefit others – in road safety, say, or the treatment of mental health or addiction services, to name but a few. And there are those who selflessly allow organ harvesting, giving new life to strangers. What a legacy.

On occasion, when I inform the police or gardaí that the postmortem findings are ambivalent but the death should be regarded as a homicide, depending on what information and evidence come to light, they are incredulous. Again, what would I have to gain? Nothing. But, as I explain to them, they will have a lot to lose if this death is not treated as a homicide – until such time as they are fully satisfied that they can find no evidence to support it. This mainly applies to deaths following head injury.

I was extremely fortunate that all of the pathologists I encountered during my training, first as a histopathologist and then as a forensic pathologist, were not only exceptional in their work but had integrity and, most importantly, bucket loads of common sense: no flights of fancy here, hard facts and a scientific appraisal of them, leading to a considered opinion – accident, suicide or homicide. I am proud to have been accepted into that fold.

Rod Burnett, my first boss, introduced me to the concept of Occam's Razor, 'The simplest solution is most likely the right one', and that if there are competing hypotheses that make the same prediction, select the one with the fewest assumptions. That is forensic pathology in a nutshell. Another saying in Ireland is 'It is what it is.' Exactly. I despair of pathologists who try to make cases into something they're not, usually the murder that never was. I may not be the sharpest scalpel in the pathology fraternity but I have plenty of common sense, a very underrated attribute.

When considering the manner of death – accident, suicide or homicide – once the autopsy is complete, I first consider a simple explanation for the injuries I have found. Can I find an explanation for this death other than murder? Only once I have no other alternative for an injury, or a series of injuries, will I confidently report it as homicide.

The body and its tissues have a limited response to any insult, particularly trauma, and therefore there may be many different mechanisms of injury with the same outcome. In simple terms, a bruise can be caused in a fall, or by a punch, a kick, being struck by an object or bumped into in a football game or— Well, the list is endless. In court I have heard believable and unbelievable explanations for each and every injury I have described on a body. But remember Occam's Razor. Is there one simple explanation for them all? To make sense of the findings I must marry the outside, or surface, trauma with the internal damage. Forensic pathology is a problem-solving speciality, and this is the greatest problem to be solved: murder or not. No prizes for a correct answer. The possibility of being struck off the medical register for a wrong one. No pressure, then!

Deaths due to head injuries are always problematic. Blunt-force head injuries are common. Around a million persons a year in the UK present at A&E with a head injury, ranging from trivial to catastrophic. Particularly when it comes to children, parents and carers are not going to take any chances. Only about 10 per cent of these will be admitted, many just for overnight observation, but in those with more significant injuries, such as a skull fracture, admission means that, should their condition deteriorate, there will be immediate medical assistance, which should limit ongoing brain damage and prevent secondary complications. Around 5 per cent of those admitted will be referred for a neurological opinion, in some instances with a view to neurosurgical intervention.

Strict criteria apply to those referred for surgical

treatment, usually to excavate a blood clot or remove a foreign body in penetrating injuries, such as gunshot wounds. One of the predictors of any head injury is the level of coma at the time of presentation. This is measured by the Glasgow Coma Scale, which measures activity of the brain. Full consciousness scores fifteen and the lowest score is three; where you are on this scale will determine your prognosis and whether or not surgery will be of any benefit. Age is also a factor: young injured will always get the benefit of the doubt. Head injuries are one of the commonest causes of death in young adults in developed countries.

Of the five thousand with severe head injuries in the UK each year, some will not survive and many survivors will have a degree of permanent brain damage. This will range from memory loss to a physical disability or epilepsy.

In general, a head injury causes death because of either injury to the brain or haemorrhage. There may be extensive bruising and tearing of the brain tissue and bleeding into the brain caused by severe trauma, such as a fall from a height, a road traffic incident or even a gunshot wound, the damage so severe that the brain can no longer function. The majority of lethal head injuries show extensive, and often disfiguring, injuries to the face and scalp, complex and comminuted fractures of the skull, bleeding around and into the brain and devastating injury to the brain. There is no doubt that death is due to a head injury.

However, not all deaths due to head trauma are as simple to reconcile with the circumstances. These are often associated with people found collapsed, or dead, little known about their movements in the few days leading up to their death, and the type of injury, which could have been caused accidentally or been deliberately inflicted.

There may be a laceration (or lacerations) caused by a fall or blow (or blows) to the head, which haemorrhages. The scalp has a rich network of blood vessels and crushing it may cause the tissues to rupture, tearing the vessels, which bleed profusely, to the extent that, if no medical treatment is sought, death can occur. There are several such deaths every year. Usually drink is involved and the majority are accidental head injuries, falling over drunk. Unfortunately, drink clouds the judgement, which includes failing to recognise that you have sustained a potentially fatal injury.

The scene holds the clue to this being the cause

of death. Blood will have been trailed throughout the home, in the bathroom, where the victim may have made some attempt to clean themselves up, pools of blood on the floor where they lay after the fall and in the bed where they 'woke up' dead. Such an innocuous injury but with devastating effects.

On one occasion an elderly man was found dead outside his front door. He lived on the top floor of a tenement building. He had been out for a few drinks the night before, and was found by a neighbour going to work on a Saturday morning. The body came into the mortuary as a sudden death, most likely a heart attack given the man's age. I was not asked to see the body at the scene. Externally there was a large laceration to his head, which could have been caused if he had collapsed when he suffered a heart attack. Internally he had definite evidence of narrowing of his coronary arteries and scarring of his heart muscle, but there was no fracture of his skull, nor was there bleeding into the skull cavity or the brain. Was this a natural death or might the heart disease be a red herring and instead he had simply fallen and sustained a laceration and bled to death? Natural versus accidental death.

If the former, the scalp laceration would not be expected to bleed much, but if the latter, I would have expected copious amounts of blood where his body was discovered. I asked the policeman who had accompanied the body to the mortuary if there was much blood at the scene. 'Not much. But the police photographer was there so I'll get him to bring in the photos.'

The photographs told the complete story. The 'not much' blood was seen cascading down two flights of stairs to the entrance to the tenement close. Cause of death: haemorrhage from a head injury sustained in a fall, acute alcohol intoxication a contributory cause. In common parlance, a Friday night drunken fall. I'm sure that policeman is now a detective superintendent somewhere remote.

The bleeding from a head injury might be internal, inside the skull cavity. The skull is a rigid bony box, designed to protect the brain, which takes up most of the space inside. It is suspended in the cerebro-spinal fluid (CSF), which acts as a shock absorber. Trauma to the head, whether or not there is a skull fracture, may result in tearing of the vessels inside the skull cavity, which will bleed into the enclosed space. As the blood collects internally and begins to clot, its mass causes the pressure inside the skull to rise. The brain reacts by swelling, further increasing the pressure, leading to a deterioration in the Glasgow Coma Scale score. The powerhouse of the brain, the brainstem, is at the junction between the brain and the spinal cord, hovering just above the foramen magnum, the hole in the floor of the skull, and this is compressed as the pressure continues to rise.

This causes a power cut. The main controls of consciousness, respiration and heart function begin to shut down. The conscious level falls and the breathing becomes laboured. Without medical attention death will occur shortly after breathing ceases; with medical attention, artificial respiration will offer a stay of execution, but that might only be temporary depending on the extent of damage to the brain. The prognosis will be determined by the results of brainstem tests, which will be carried out over the course of the next few days. At best the patient may survive with minor brain injury or, at worst, they will be declared brainstem dead, with no hope for survival.

I have had calls from the police about people who have sustained a head injury in an assault and are now on life support, everyone expecting the worst. I am always uncomfortable when contemplating a postmortem examination while someone is hanging on to life. But often the call is premature. Several days later when I enquire about the injured party, I hear, 'Oh! Him! He came round and signed himself out of hospital. Says it was just an accident. Sorry, Doc, should have let you know.' Prepare for the worst but hope for the best. Still, lads, wait for the final gasp before you call me.

But, no matter the outcome, the question I have to answer is: how was the head injury caused? The majority of head injuries are accidental, so how do you separate out the potential homicidal head injuries?

Determining how a head injury was caused can be problematic, particularly if there is only one point of impact, only one area of injury, a bruise, graze or laceration. The more extensive the trauma, the easier it is to determine in what circumstances it could have been sustained. The overall pattern of injuries must be taken into consideration, not just the head trauma. Are there injuries elsewhere on the body, which could have been caused by a fall, or are there injuries that suggest an assault?

The fatal injury is obvious but the minor injuries tell the pathologist more of a story. These are the injuries overlooked by everyone else. They are of no importance because they are not life-threatening. When assault victims survive long enough to get into hospital the emphasis is on sustaining their life. The focus is on the injury (or injuries) that requires remedial treatment. Who cares about the bruises on the arms or legs? Thankfully, nurses do. Once in the ward, nurses take a more holistic approach, treating the whole person, not the injury or ailment. They have been trained to take copious notes on the state of their patients so minor marks and injuries will be described and noted.

When dealing with any injured party who has died after their admission to hospital, I always ask for the nursing notes, particularly the detailed notes from intensive care, which often include diagrams with the injuries mapped. This is important to me because after a few days of medical treatment there will have been so much handling and medical interference, and bruises due to blood-taking and injections on the arms especially. Knowing the extent of the injuries present when the person arrived in hospital will assist in determining how they sustained the significant injuries: accident, suicide or homicide.

While most head injuries are sustained accidentally, there is usually a link with alcohol.

The night starts well, then gets a wee bit rowdy as the drink kicks in. All good fun. At the end of the night everyone staggers off, heading for home. Most will make it unscathed, bar a thumping headache and queasy stomach, while others feign loss of memory rather than admit what, or who, happened the night before. Anyone who has had the misfortune to spend a Friday or Saturday night in A&E will have been subject to the antics of the inebriated few. They are often still in the 'happy' but disruptive phase, unaware that they are testing the patience of those present, staff and patients. It is the last thing you need when you're feeling very poorly.

The worst offenders may be a group of young men, accompanying one of their friends, who fell over and cracked his head on the kerb. They eventually got him to his feet. They aren't sure if he was knocked out or not. Taking him to hospital seemed the right thing to do. Unfortunately, if the group becomes belligerent, they may be shown the door, leaving their injured friend to be seen. Sometimes the injured party might decide that he, rarely she, is fine, no need to wait, and all head home.

Alcohol and head injuries are not a good

combination. From a medical point of view, the depressive effect of alcohol on the brain will mask the early signs of a head injury. If the injured person leaves before he, or she, is examined or treated, there is potential danger to their life. This is the young person found dead at home the day after a 'good' night out.

It's the classic tale of the head injury complicated by internal bleeding and the formation of the extradural haemorrhage. As the tale unfolds of the events of the fatal night, I have already made my diagnosis.

A young man's life has been snuffed out, a tragedy, but an accident with no one to blame. When the side of his head hit the kerb, the skull cracked. A skull fracture is not synonymous with death, but is an indication that the head injury is significant. It indicates that the impact was forceful. The skull is protected from the force of impact by the thickness of the hair and the scalp. Perhaps security staff would reconsider their 'hard man image' of a shaved head if they realised that lustrous locks might be to their advantage when a fight breaks out, particularly if weapons are used and there is a risk of a blow to their head.

A fracture to the side of the skull may be

complicated by bleeding into the skull cavity, as there is a fairly large artery running up the inside of the skull, just above the ear, the middle meningeal artery, which may be torn when the bone breaks. This diagnosis cannot be made by simply examining the person, but requires an X-ray to show the fracture or a scan to pick up early bleeding. Immediately after sustaining the injury, the victim will usually exhibit no signs or symptoms but, over a period of hours, the torn blood vessel will leak into the skull cavity, directly between the bone and the tough tissue, the dura, which lines the skull, hence its description as extradural. As the bleeding continues, the pressure inside the skull increases, as does the pressure on the brainstem. This causes a decrease in the conscious level.

A major complication is that as the injured party had been drinking and had obviously shown evidence of the depressive effects of alcohol, before and after the fall, it is difficult to identify when the blood clot in the skull reaches a critical volume and begins to cause symptoms, unless the person is being monitored by medical personnel in hospital. Even that is not fool-proof as people may deteriorate so rapidly that the danger to their life is not recognised in time. If an extradural haemorrhage is diagnosed, it is amenable to surgical treatment and, as it often occurs without any significant brain injury, a full recovery can be expected.

Sometimes life is not that simple. While the majority of deaths caused by an extradural haemorrhage are accidental, the investigation of the death would have had a different outcome if the deceased had been involved in a minor fracas, something as simple as a bit of pushing and shoving, larking about as young lads do, especially if drink is involved. Accident becomes a potential homicide. The cause of death remains the same but the circumstances are different. That is a matter for the police, not the pathologist.

If an extradural haemorrhage is fairly straightforward to investigate, another intracranial haemorrhage is anything but: the subdural haemorrhage. In this instance the bleeding inside the skull cavity, while also due to head trauma, occurs in different circumstances. This type of injury is more commonly associated with relatively minor head injuries in the elderly, chronic drinkers and anyone who has loss of brain tissue. The brain is suspended in the cerebrospinal fluid and small vessels run between the brain and the lining of the skull: the bridging veins, so-called because they bridge the gap between the brain and the dura. When the brain shrinks, the tension on them increases, and so does the risk of the vessels snapping when the head accelerates rapidly or the brain is caused to reverberate due to a minor impact on the head. The small bridging vessels are low-pressure veins, and when they are torn, they bleed slowly in the space around the brain, which is greater than normal due to the smaller brain taking up less space in the skull cavity. In contrast with the torn artery causing an extradural bleed, it will take some considerable time for the blood collecting inside the skull in the subdural space to be of sufficient volume to cause the intracranial pressure to rise and symptoms to develop. This may take a day or two, sometimes weeks. Even when the injured person begins to show signs and symptoms, the underlying cause may not be recognised, the change in their actions or personality thought to be related to their underlying neurological condition.

The diagnosis will be made only if they are subject to a scan. But sometimes it is only established postmortem. The difficulty is how the subdural haemorrhage was caused. Was there a single incident? And, if so, when did it happen? Was it the result of a fall, or falls, or could they have been pushed or struck by a third party? This is a vulnerable population: the elderly may be unsteady on their feet and prone to falls or they may be being abused; those living with dementia are similarly at risk; chronic alcoholics may fall when intoxicated and may be subject to violent behaviour, whether or not they are the instigator. So, a major difficulty is accident versus homicide. But even if there is evidence of a violent incident, during which the deceased received a head injury, there may be a difficulty with the time frame. Subdurals take time to develop and there is usually no close temporal relationship between a specific incident and a symptomatic subdural haemorrhage. There is always the possibility of sustaining another head injury shortly before or after. These deaths fall into the 'I'm not 100 per cent sure' category. Accident? Maybe. Homicide? Maybe.

Often it comes down to the pattern of trauma. Are all the injuries relatively minor? Are they due to a fall or falls? Or might some injuries have been inflicted by a third party? Is there evidence of rough handling or injuries that might indicate an attempt at self-defence? Into the latter category fall the injuries to 'protected' areas of the body, such as a black eye or gripping injuries on the inside of the upper arms. These raise a red flag to the pathologist. It may be that there is a simple explanation for the fatal head injury, but the investigating officers cannot take a chance and will continue until all lines of enquiry are exhausted.

In the 1970s and 1980s the neuropathology department in Glasgow, which no longer exists, had a world-class reputation. The research carried out by Professors Adams and Graham helped to discover why some victims of road traffic accidents and assaults, who had sustained a head injury but had no discernible injury to the brain or bleeding around it, remained comatose. They were instrumental in describing the pathological condition diffuse axonal injury (DAI). This is an injury at a cellular level, which could only be diagnosed after death by examining the brain. Their research also identified the mechanism of trauma, rapid acceleration, and/or sudden deceleration. The forces produced in certain conditions were shown to be sufficient to snap the long tendrils, the axons, which transmit information from the nucleus of the nerve cells, the neurones in the brain. The extent of this trauma may be so devastating that death follows rapidly, but if the injury is less severe, some recovery is possible. The sensitivity of scans is now such that the diagnosis can be made in life. But there is still no treatment for this type of brain injury and, if the brainstem is at least partly spared, the injured party may remain comatose indefinitely, or at least while the other major organs continue functioning.

I was extremely fortunate to have known and worked with the two men. When I entered forensic pathology there was still work to be done and it was exciting to be party to their discovery that diffuse axonal injury could be caused by a simple fall – someone fell to the ground without being pushed or propelled with force. Prior to that, if the cause of a person's coma was DAI, the death was treated as a potential homicide. Now we can accept that such a head injury may have been sustained accidentally.

You cannot make an omelette without breaking eggs and so it was with research at that time. Organs were retained and sent to specialists, most commonly cardiac pathologists and neuropathologists. When someone dies in hospital after a long illness, they have usually been subject to extensive investigations. The medical staff know how every cell is functioning, or not. A diagnosis has been made. There are no questions left unanswered. Death is not a surprise but an expected event, even if it was unwelcome. But when death is sudden and unexpected, or the cause undetermined, there will always be questions to answer. Before the sophisticated technology now available to the medical profession existed, the diagnostic tools were relatively basic, even if the hands that held them were far from 'basic'.

Deaths in these circumstances have to be reported to the coroner, or the procurator fiscal, who authorises the pathologist to determine the cause of death. This might include consultation with another expert and removal of an organ for further examination by a specialist. As these deaths are investigated by the coroner, or procurator fiscal, the family are not consulted and their consent to retain an organ is not required. But the families should be notified if an organ has been retained.

Over years these experts beavered away, trying to unlock the mysteries of the heart and the brain. When they had a viable theory, they sometimes had to resort to animal experiments to test it. Such experimental work is no longer condoned in medical circles but in those days it helped us understand the mechanics of failure of the heart and brain, in neuropathology particularly the brain's reaction to trauma. It was unfortunate that animals were sacrificed, but at that time technology was not sophisticated enough to progress these fields of medicine. Medicine today is very different. There has been much talk that the role of the pathologist, and even the forensic pathologist, will be usurped by scanning machines. Perhaps the same could be said for any doctor. Should we just have banks of scanners and move people through on conveyor belts? Why bother with a cervical smear if you could just pop into the scanner? You don't even have to take your clothes off. We're not there yet.

In the early days of research into the effects of trauma on the brain, the putative diagnosis of DAI could only be confirmed after death and required a thorough examination of the brain. This type of examination takes weeks. The brain has to be fixed in formalin, slivers of tissue cut and stained with specific dyes, but it meant we could now explain to families what had happened and why the injured person would never have woken up. At that time, and even today, the pathologist can retain organs and tissues taken at the time of the postmortem for further examination if it is thought this will assist in determining the cause of death.

Unfortunately, many people are not aware of this, and there was an outcry when it came to light in England that some families had not known about the retention of organs in baby deaths. This has led to a change in practices throughout the UK and Ireland and now families are fully informed about organ retention. They will then have the choice of what happens to the organ when all the investigations are complete: its return for burial or cremation; or similar disposal by the pathology department. In Dublin there is a garden of remembrance for organs cremated by the Office of the State Pathologist.

I only ever retained an organ if it was entirely necessary. Having received a first-class education in trauma neuropathology in Glasgow, I rarely needed to retain a brain. The difficult cases are those who die rapidly, within a few minutes, with a relatively minor head injury and apparent minimal gross injury to the brain. In the older age group this is usually because of intercurrent heart disease, a stress-associated heart attack. But how do we explain the suddenness of death in younger, supposedly healthy individuals? There is still so much that we do not know and cannot fully explain. In such deaths the forensic pathologist will proffer an opinion based on the postmortem findings and current medical thinking. This is by no means absolute and we all accept that there may be alternative explanations.

One such case was the death of a young man, Brian Murphy, in 2000. A fight had broken out outside Annabel's nightclub in Dublin city centre. Several young men were involved but Brian died in the incident. There were accounts of what had happened, who had done what, and four of the young men involved were charged with offences related to the assault leading to Brian's death. Professor Harbison, the state pathologist, carried out the postmortem. He concluded that Brian's death was due to head trauma. The case came to court and one young man was found guilty of manslaughter and sentenced to four years in prison. His counsel lodged an appeal against his conviction, which was successfully overturned, the conviction deemed unsafe. By this time, Professor Harbison had retired so, when the DPP was considering a retrial, I was asked to review the postmortem photographs and provide a report.

Brian had died at the scene, despite extensive attempts by the paramedics to resuscitate him. The photographs showed some injuries to the head but there was no skull fracture or bleeding into the skull cavity. The brain was swollen but not bruised or torn. He appeared to have been otherwise healthy: there was no obvious natural disease that could have caused sudden death. He had been drinking but not excessively. Brian died in the assault, but what was the mechanism?

Brain swelling is a reaction to any insult to the brain; when due to trauma it is not usually so rapid in onset or so extreme. The most common cause of brain swelling is hypoxia, a lack of oxygen. But why? Potentially fatal brain swelling can complicate even minor head trauma in young children, but not in this age group. Why else would he be deprived of oxygen? Blockage of the airways is a possibility if there were injuries to the nose or mouth and blood tracks down into the trachea, preventing air getting into the lungs. That would have been evident as blood in the trachea and haemorrhages in the lungs, but neither was present. Something had affected the respiratory mechanism. In all complex cases a second, third or even fourth opinion will be sought. I discussed the case with my colleague and then I delved into the literature.

In forensic pathology in the UK and Ireland

little meaningful research is carried out. This is not due to apathy: the system precludes it. Most forensic pathologists have large caseloads and are stretched to the limits, leaving little or no time for teaching and research. In relative terms, the forensic population is small in comparison to that of the USA, so we are dependent on the research carried out by our American colleagues, which has far more weight behind it.

In forensic circles there is a dynasty of forensic pathologists, the Di Maios, father and son. They have written the reference books we use and their research is renowned. Vincent Di Maio, among others, cited that in some head injuries deaths are due to 'post-traumatic apnoea', the breathing stopping for long enough that the brain is irreparably damaged. This was said to have been recognised in concussive head injuries, in particular. Holding of breath after a head injury is common, but usually only for a few seconds. Why should the period of apnoea be prolonged in some cases?

Di Maio postulated that animal experiments had shown that if alcohol was given to a dog before it was injured the period of apnoea was prolonged. Such experiments cannot be carried out on humans so we are reliant on animal models for an answer.

Armed with this information, I tried to explain to the DPP what I thought might have happened to Brian Murphy and how the assault had caused his death. Brian Murphy went out on a Wednesday night: there was no reason at all why he should not have returned home safe and sound. He had a few drinks but that would not have been expected to cause his death, even if he was a novice drinker. But on that night Brian died. The only variable was an incident during which he was assaulted. Had that not happened he would not have died.

I explained my opinion as to the sequence of events on that fateful night. The DPP took all of the available evidence into consideration and decided not to pursue a retrial. As a result, I was not required to give evidence in court. My report was leaked to the media and some assumed that it was on the basis of the report that the DPP had decided not to proceed. Highly improbable: the bottom line was that Brian Murphy had died after being injured in an assault. The DPP has never, to my knowledge, made a decision on whether or not to proceed with a case based on my evidence alone.

The press made much of the case collapsing and

rich boys getting off scot-free after causing the death of a young man. I was shocked when it was reported that I was alleged to have implied that, as Brian had been drinking, he brought about his own demise. No. That was not the case.

Suddenly everyone had an opinion on this. The constant posturing by some and the press coverage must have been terrible for Brian's family to deal with, on top of the realisation that those they had thought responsible for their son's death would not have to account for their actions. This is the hardest part of my job, seeing the disappointment of parents when they have lost a child and feel that those involved in the investigation of the death have somehow let them down. I wish there was a magic wand to right all the wrongs in the world but there isn't. We mere mortals all strive to do our best, and I'm sorry that sometimes it isn't enough. If only the press had awaited the outcome of the inquest. The jury returned a verdict of unlawful killing.

While head injuries continue to confound the forensic pathologist, sharp and gunshot injuries are more straightforward. There are no nuances:

the injuries are obvious and deadly. However, with these deaths there is the added possibility of self-inflicted injuries: accident, homicide or suicide.

In Scotland, as most murders were stabbings, the police assumed that death from a stab wound, or wounds, was a homicide unless there was strong evidence to the contrary. Of course, as I have said, I start with the premise that there is a simple explanation and only when that has been excluded will I agree that a death is a homicide. In my early days, homicide deaths due to a single stab wound were not uncommon, although often the injuries were multiple – in some cases in excess of a hundred. But the number of stab wounds is not the determining factor in deciding the manner of death.

When there is a single stab wound, the death could have been accidental, homicidal or suicidal. The first deciding factor is the site of the injury: is it in an accessible site? People do not stab themselves in the back. Next, are there other injuries, minor, non-fatal stab or incised wounds? If so, where are they on the body and could they have been self-inflicted or have resulted from a struggle, the so-called defence injuries? The self-inflicted injuries of a suicide attempt tend to be on the front of the wrist, fairly regular, multiple and shallow: the tentative injuries. In contrast, defence injuries are on the palms or backs of the hands and on the back and sides of the arms. They vary in length, depth and direction.

When there is a single stab wound the site and appearance are important but so also are the depth and direction of internal track: upwards, downwards or diagonally through the tissues and organs. The dimensions of the wound through the skin will give an indication of the size and type of knife used. Of course, if this was a self-inflicted injury, or injuries, the knife used should have been present at the scene. Multiple stab wounds do not exclude self-infliction. Such injuries tend to be clustered together on the left side of the chest, over the heart area. They tend to vary from pinpricks to large, gaping wounds, shallow to deeply penetrating; one or more will have wounded the heart, lung or a major vessel. More than one knife may have been used.

Homicidal stabbings tend to be less precise. They are dynamic situations so the wounds will be anywhere on the body, front, back, sides, arms and legs, depending which area was accessible to the perpetrator, or perpetrators. If the dimensions of the wounds suggest that the injuries were inflicted by more than one knife, there may have been more than one attacker. If there are clusters of knife injuries, this suggests that the victim was unable to move, possibly due to injuries already inflicted or they were trapped. Incised wounds to the face may be inflicted in the course of a knife assault and while some may have been random slashes during the course of the melee, marking of the face is a deliberate action to disfigure the victim. The worst injuries are those to the hands caused by trying to grasp the blade. They express the terror and the struggle that the lifeless body does not convey. Dead men do tell tales.

Accidental sharp injuries occur, but usually the scene is key in such deaths. Many may be work-related – the victim is impaled on some equipment or machinery. Occasionally they may be drink-related, such as a fall through a glass door or even the incised wound caused by the broken glass or bottle. The injuries tend to be haphazard and death is often due to blood lost from slicing through an artery rather than piercing an internal organ.

It still amazes me that defence counsel will proffer a defence of 'semi-accidental' injury in a fatal stabbing. 'My client was standing at the bus stop, with a knife in his hand [whittling, or cleaning his nails, I presume] when a man unexpectedly launched himself at him/ran into him and impaled himself on my client's knife.' My heavens, wouldn't that be a shock when you were waiting patiently for the number 41 to Swords?

I guess I, too, would be mighty miffed at being charged with murder in those circumstances. But this is the central criminal court, and I have sworn to tell the truth. It is no place for levity and, as an unbiased witness, I must consider all propositions, even if I think they are preposterous. It will be for the jury to decide whether or not this was a likely scenario. My role is to consider whether or not a certain action, or actions, could result in the pattern of wounding I observed at postmortem. Accident versus homicide.

My response to the court when considering the account of an incident from the accused's point of view will depend on the number, site and direction of the fatal injury, or injuries, present. I must consider only whether it is possible to replicate the injury in the manner described. If there is a single stab wound, the site and direction of the internal track will enable the pathologist to determine the position of the two parties in relation to one another and even how the knife was held. Could two bodies colliding in the manner described replicate the fatal injury? If so, the answer is 'Yes, that injury could have been caused in such a manner.' Raised eyebrow! We always add caveats, such as the knife being held firmly, or it would have been deflected, and it would have had to be sharp. However, we have to accept the laws of physics and agree that the opposing forces of the colliding bodies are additive. But, even then, would the combined forces be sufficient for penetration of the blade? That question I could not answer.

There was precious little in the literature regarding the dynamics of stab incidents. Professor Bernard Knight has carried out some experimentation on the force required for a knife to penetrate a body, and this was replicated by his successors, but the equipment was rudimentary and the results unreliable. Normally I would look to our American counterparts for reference material, but they have carried out little research on stab incidents. The biggest problem in the States is gun crime.

In order to test the accidental impaling, or 'run on', hypothesis in those cases with a single wound, my colleague Mike Curtis and I approached the mechanical engineering department at University College Dublin (UCD). The head of department, Professor Michael Gilchrist, was fascinated by our 'problem', and for the next few years one of his students researched how we could quantify the force required to penetrate the skin and internal tissues. The result of extensive experimental work was a formula that could be used to determine the force required for any knife to penetrate. This, of course, had to be explained to us in simplistic terms. We certainly were not the sharpest knives in the drawer.

Be careful what you wish for: if we couldn't grasp the mathematics, how could we explain it to a jury? Nevertheless, this research confirmed what we had already suspected, that the main factor determining the force required for penetration of a body was the shape, angle and sharpness of the tip of a blade: steak knives were the most efficient. The clue is in the name – essentially, we are meat. A more surprising finding was that, with a sharp knife, relatively little force is required to penetrate the skin and cause a fatal injury: the tip of a knife indents the skin and, if sharp, will pierce it with little effort, and thereafter the blade will glide smoothly through the tissues, unless it meets bone or cartilage. The 'run on' scenario of two bodies colliding cannot be dismissed out of hand.

There are few opportunities to carry out research in forensic pathology. Unlike trials of drugs and novel medical procedures intended to improve health and prolong life, the bottom line with forensic pathology is death. Volunteers for our trials would be few and far between, and ethics committees would be reluctant to allow any such research. So, all of the research the Office of the State Pathologist has carried out to date has been on material legitimately procured from a butcher, mainly pig carcasses and pig skin: close to human skin and tissue, but not identical. Better than nothing. At least we are getting closer to having valid scientific evidence to support certain hypotheses and theories. The 'showman' forensic pathologist of past times has been usurped by a less dogmatic breed. Almost.

In the UK and Ireland, guns have not reached epidemic proportions – yet – but not for want of trying on the part of our villainous population. In Ireland, shotguns can be accessed easily, but they are rather bulky, useful if the intention is to frighten, but not if you're trying to keep under garda radar. In recent years there appears to have been a steady stream of handguns coming in from Eastern Europe – hence the increasing number of gunshot deaths. In comparison, Scottish gangsters seem reluctant to fully embrace new weaponry, sticking instead to time-honoured knives and blunt instruments. If it ain't broke, don't fix it . . .

Shotguns are more likely to be the weapon of choice for suicide attempts in the UK and Ireland because they are more readily available. But that is not to say that people shouldn't have access to guns because they might use them to kill themselves: that is just the method of choice. Suicide is not about availability of guns, drugs, or whatever: it's about something else completely, a symptom of despair and depression none of us wants to experience. I find it especially sad when the person is elderly, usually living alone. Could anything have been done to prevent their death? No. But perhaps we should be less wrapped up in our own little worlds, and the virtual world created by technology, and stop, look up and say hello. It might make someone's day.

The issue with shotguns is that they cause devastating injuries at close range. It is easy to see how those injuries cause death, but are we dealing with an accident, suicide or homicide? As the distance between gun and target increases, the pellets fan out and their lethality diminishes. And, of course, as distance increases, the likelihood of a third party firing the shotgun increases, particularly when out of the victim's arm's length.

Suicide deaths are not a diagnostic problem: there is a predilection for specific sites of injury that the forensic pathologist recognises. The background history and the scene examination fill in the blanks. But suicide still holds stigma in some sections of the community, particularly in Ireland. Sometimes, with the best of intentions, families may alter the scene by removing the gun. Instead of having the desired effect of fooling us into thinking the death is due to something else, a heart attack perhaps, if we find that someone has died from a gunshot injury and there was no gun at the scene, the death becomes a potential homicide, with all that that entails. The neighbours need never have known what happened but they will now because the gardaí will question everyone within earshot of a gun blast. Please, resist the temptation to meddle.

In one case, an elderly man was found by his nephew, a shotgun on the floor. He lifted it and put it into the gun 'cupboard', actually the wardrobe, while he was waiting for the police to arrive. His uncle had a long history of heart disease so it was perfectly reasonable to assume his death was due to natural causes. A local GP was called to confirm the death. He noted a large hole in the abdomen but thought this might be due to him having died a day or so before his body was discovered. In the mortuary the APT was more concerned. I confirmed that death was due to a shotgun injury and was consistent with self-infliction, as long as the gun had been nearby. The nephew apologised: he had thought his uncle had been careless in leaving the gun lying around. We gave him the benefit of the doubt.

In a similar case a mother hid the gun her son had used. His death was treated as sudden and unexpected, and the pathologist carrying out the postmortem was perplexed that he couldn't find a cause of death. He noted a tiny hole in the side of the head and wondered if the young man might have hit it on the corner of a chest of drawers when he collapsed. We discussed the case on the phone. 'No, no obvious cause of death': the only abnormality was the small injury at the side of the head. He said there was a tiny crack in the skull but no trauma to the brain, so he had no reason to suspect that this injury had killed the man. 'X-ray the brain,' I said.

An hour later he phoned back to report a pellet had been found in it. Unusual, but as I had expected, he had been shot. By whom? A search of the house revealed nothing out of the ordinary. On further questioning the mother reached into her bag and pulled out an air pistol. In an effort to avoid the shame of the act, she had advertised the fact to the whole neighbourhood. They had the good grace to rally around her. People are not that judgemental. There but for the grace of God . . .

Shotguns in the wrong hands can be lethal. Careless handling may result in accidental injuries, even in experienced gunmen. The site of the injury and a description of the circumstances are usually sufficient to confirm that the injury, fatal or not, was accidentally inflicted by the person with the gun or a 'friend'. In one instance a couple of 'hard men' were on their way to commit some crime, armed with a loaded shotgun. One, literally riding shotgun, was sitting in the front passenger seat, the butt of the gun on the floor between his feet, his chin resting on the muzzle. There is a television programme that shows clips of people doing extremely stupid things, which the audience can see are not going to end well. Well, I'm sure you're one step ahead of our hapless criminal. The car went down a pothole and the gun went off. Hapless became headless. The driver panicked – wouldn't you? – and bolted. An 'accidental' death.

Shotguns are deliberately lethal in the hands of the criminal fraternity. They are still used in robberies – the intention is probably to intimidate, but when the going gets rough, the gun may be fired. During an armed raid a security guard was shot in the back and died on the way to hospital. There was no doubt: death was due to a shotgun wound to the back of his chest and the pellets had shredded his internal organs. What was of interest was that while the entry wound on his back was the typical large hole expected, it was surrounded by the imprint of the gun's muzzle, which had the appearance of a figure of eight. The shotgun had two barrels and one had been discharged when the gun was pushed into his back. The men responsible for the robbery had worn balaclavas. Identification was difficult, but fingerprints found on a vehicle at the scene led to one man being arrested.

He pleaded not guilty – 'Wasn't there, wasn't me.' Rather than sit down and shut up, the defence team decided on damage limitation. Their client wasn't responsible but, anyway, wasn't it likely that the death had been accidental in the melee of the raid. Accident versus homicide. No, a shotgun was discharged directly into the back of the deceased and the gun was firmly against his back when the trigger was pulled. Homicide.

The jury heard all the evidence and returned a verdict of not proven. The defence had challenged the fingerprint evidence, which the prosecution stated put the accused at the scene, and therefore possibly with the offending gun in his hand, but the forensic scientist agreed he could not determine when the fingerprint was left on the vehicle. It might have been left at another time.

Another case began when the fire brigade received a panicked phone call from a woman who said that the cottage next door was in flames. An elderly man and his ill wife lived there, with their two dogs, and hadn't been seen in the last couple of days. The fire was raging when the fire brigade arrived, the roof already partly collapsed. If anyone was inside it was too late to save them. Eventually, the flames were brought under control sufficiently for a fireman to get inside safely.

In what appeared to have been the bedroom two bodies were found, one on the remains of a bed, the other as if seated on a chair. A tragic accident: the cause of the fire would be uncovered later when the scene was examined by the experts. The bodies were taken to the local mortuary for examination. Unfortunately, they were burned beyond recognition, so identification would be a major problem. Non-forensic pathologists balk at having to deal with fire deaths as they are of the opinion that a postmortem is futile, but those of us in the know can get blood out of the proverbial stone and will be able to identify the body or bodies and determine whether or not they had died from the fire.

The pathologist, mindful of the potential difficulties, requested the radiology department to take X-rays of the bodies. X-rays were taken, and the radiologist phoned the pathologist: there appeared to be small pieces of metal in the heads, probably just debris, but they looked a bit like shotgun pellets. The pathologist phoned the police superintendent. He reassured the pathologist that the remains of a shotgun had been found in the bedroom so there had probably been cartridges as well: nothing to worry about.

Except he was worried enough to call me. He just wanted to run it by me, there was no need for me to do anything – the postmortem would be carried out on Monday and all would be well. But this was Friday night. Nearly three days before there would be a definitive answer. The radiologist had thought the metal could be shotgun pellets, and that they were limited to the heads troubled me greatly. At best it was a red herring, but we could have a suicide pact, a murder-suicide or, at worst, a double murder.

I asked him to describe the scene in detail. He added one new piece of information: the couple's dogs had been found dead under the chair on which their master had been sitting. Dogs will go berserk in a fire, not sleep through it. 'Humour me! Ask the local vet to X-ray the dogs.'

Later that night he got back to me: 'The vet thinks they've been shot.' That clinched the deal. I did the postmortems the next morning. The bodies were badly damaged by the fire so identification would be difficult but not impossible. The destruction of the heads meant that had X-rays not been taken an unwary pathologist might have put down all the damage to the fire. It soon became apparent that both victims had been shot in the head. Apart from the pellets scattered through what was left of the brains there was a gaping hole in the side of the female's head and a shotgun entry wound through the roof of the male's mouth. I had no doubt that his injury was self-inflicted, but hers had been caused by a third party: her husband.

Although fire had ravaged the bodies, I was still able to identify the bottom part of the windpipe in both. There was no blackening of the lining, so neither had breathed in smoke: both were dead by the time the fire had started. I was also able to get enough blood for toxicological analyses, which confirmed that they had not breathed in fumes – the carbon monoxide level was within normal limits in both parties and there was no evidence of drink or drugs. Still, was it possible that the man could have shot his wife, the dogs and himself and been able to set the house on fire to cover his tracks? The fire investigators were able to show that the fire had started in the bedroom and that it had been deliberately set. Once the fire was started he could have sat in the chair and shot himself.

If the call for emergency services had come a few hours later all traces of the actual cause of death would have been lost. This would have been another statistic: two fatalities in a house fire. But we had uncovered the truth – well, the stark facts. Was this a final act of love or of desperation? We'll never know. How would you react if the love of your life was terminally ill and you couldn't envisage life without him or her?

A woman is shot by her husband. There is a single shotgun injury to her chest, fired at close range; the plastic cup containing the pellets is found inside her chest. He admits to killing his wife but says it was an accident. A story unfolds. The teenage son found a bag containing a shotgun and some ammunition, as you do, and brought it home to show his dad. The family are in the kitchen. Daddy takes the gun, snaps it shut and pulls the trigger. Mummy is at the fridge, a foot or so away, and gets the full blast of the shot to the side of her chest. She is dead by the time the ambulance arrives.

The family are not 'gangsters' but have had a few run-ins with the police over petty thieving and drugs, father and son. There is no history of domestic violence, but that is no indicator that all in their world is rosy. The husband is charged with his wife's murder and evidence is gathered for the court case. The only sticking point is that the prosecution do not believe the husband's version of events: no one would be stupid enough to pick up a gun and pull the trigger without checking to see if it was loaded.

But, as I have learned, people do the stupidest things. Even supposedly intelligent people. At that time in Glasgow, I was a senior lecturer in the forensic medicine department and routinely lectured to medical, law and science students. One session dealt with firearms and firearm injuries. I am not a ballistics expert so I relied on the police to deliver lectures on weaponry, guns and ammunition. They would often bring along shotguns and handguns to illustrate their talk. Students, usually men, would clamour to get their hands on the decommissioned weapons, which they would gleefully point at one another, and 'fire'. Having witnessed this on previous occasions, I invited the barristers involved in the case to sit in on the firearms lecture. I reckoned that if they saw intelligent students acting in such a manner it was feasible that the husband had shot his wife accidentally. He was given the benefit of the doubt. The charge was dropped from murder to manslaughter.

Fatalities due to rifled weapons, particularly homicides, are more common now as access to handguns has become easier for the criminal fraternity. The numbers would be greater if those wielding the gun had any real idea of what they were doing. It would appear that the only instructions they hear are 'Point and shoot.' This can have dire consequences for innocent parties within a few metres of the intended target, usually a rival gang member.

In stark contrast, suicide by rifled weapon is usually the method chosen by those who have legitimate access to handguns and are used to handling them.

There is a well-recognised phenomenon described in the States as 'suicide by cop', whereby a person deliberately incites the police to shoot them. Thankfully, as the majority of police in the UK and Ireland are unarmed, this has not been adopted on these islands. I have dealt with a couple of cases in which someone has been acting strangely, drawing the attention of police to them and resulting in a car chase. On one occasion this ended with that person being shot dead. Just possibly their actions were deliberately orchestrated to provoke such a reaction. But there is no way to prove it.

Rifled weapons are lethal due to the massive energy dissipated to the internal organs when a bullet whizzes through a body. In contrast to the large entry hole caused by the mass of pellets from a shotgun, the tiny hole in the skin caused by a bullet belies the extent of the internal trauma. The energy is equated by the weight of the bullet, minimal, and the square of the speed it is travelling, considerable. The bullet from a handgun travels at 400 miles per hour and triple that from a rifle. Ramp it up to military-style weaponry and just imagine the devastation that can be caused.

The lucky few are injured and survive, usually because the bullet did not hit any vital structure but, by and large, most of us present a large target, not easy to miss. In general, in the UK and Ireland, bullets are fired indiscriminately at the intended target in the hope that some will strike the person, somewhere, anywhere. Only when the shooter is satisfied that the victim is down and out will they venture near enough to discharge a bullet into the head, the assassin's shot. There is rarely any doubt that this is a gangland-style shooting.

So, what can the pathologist add that might assist the investigating team? I rely on the police experts to identify weaponry and ammunition. As I've said, shotguns make big holes and bullets little holes, but there is more to it than that. I can assist with the range and relative positions of the parties at the moment triggers were pulled. I can retrieve a bullet from the body, which the ballistics experts can examine: the marks made on it as it travelled through the barrel of the gun are useful in identifying the weapon from which the bullet was fired and whether or not this crime is linked to previous shooting incidents with the same gun.

For range, I rely on the other products of combustion of the gunpowder, the explosion of which propels the bullet down the barrel and onwards towards its target. The flame, smoke and some unburned powder, which accompanies the bullet out, travel centimetres to a few metres at most, so if they hit the target, in this case the intended victim, I can use their presence to give the police a rough guide as to how close the shooter was to his target. Sometimes it is hard to see these on the clothes so the forensic scientists will check this for us if required.

Next, the dynamics of the situation. Bodies may be left where they fell, particularly if this was a shooting in a public place or a drive-by. But sometimes bodies will be taken and dumped elsewhere or found in burned-out cars. Were they shot while in the car or were the bodies put into a car, which was then set alight as a means to destroy evidence? To assist with this part of the inquiry, I need to determine how many bullets struck, and at what angle. In the past this was a fishing exercise but nowadays technology can assist: the body is X-rayed or scanned. X-rays will show bones fractured and any bullets still inside, but scans may also show the track of the bullet through the soft tissues. But you still need the pathologist to retrieve the bullets and interpret the injuries. The shot in the back versus the face-to-face assault: the differing trajectories of bullets through the body hold the key to the actual event. Even with X-rays bullets can be tricky.

A basic principle has it that if there is an even number of gunshot holes it is possible that all the bullets went in and out. Ah! If only it was so simple. Bullet fragments and spicules of bone exit the body. Bullets may be lodged in bone or lying free in the body cavities or even in the clothing. When there are multiple gunshot injuries it can be difficult to match up entries and exits, especially when there is massive destruction of the internal organs. Does that matter? Maybe not.

There has been an increase in drive-by shootings, with no apparent regard as to whether or not the shooting is witnessed or to the safety of innocent bystanders. There may be eye-witness accounts, but as the victim is left where they drop, we can usually piece it together. However, there may be a deliberate attempt to conceal the death, dumping the body in a location remote from the crime scene or in a vehicle, which is then set alight. Then it is important that we get as much information as possible to reconstruct the shooting incident as accurately as we can, pathologist, ballistics expert and forensic scientist collaborating. Teamwork is the key.

By determining where a bullet entered and its path through the body, I can assist in piecing together the events on that fateful day. When I had reconstructed the shooting of George Hall, the man found in the sewage works, in the pub where it had happened, I could determine that the first shot was distant, to his chest, the final shot close up, to his head. When two bodies were found in the boot of an abandoned car, both having been shot a couple of times to the body and once to the head, the sites and directions of the gunshots confirmed that one had been in the driver's seat, the other beside him when they were ambushed and shot by two gunmen.

If there is any consolation to be had, shooting incidents in the UK and Ireland are usually targeted, often gangland hits, unlike the sporadic shootings in the USA where troubled or vengeful youths vent their spleen on schools, the fatalities many but the victims arbitrarily selected. In England there was the Hungerford mass shooting in 1987, and in Scotland, Dunblane.

In March 1996, shortly after school had commenced for the day, a man armed with four handguns walked into Dunblane Primary School. Within five minutes he was dead, having shot himself after massacring sixteen five-year-olds and a teacher, as well as seriously injuring another fifteen small children. The local hospital was put on alert to receive the injured children. The staff immediately sprang into action. Word was filtering out that some children had been killed. Dunblane is a relatively small town and it was highly likely that some of the hospital staff would be connected to the children being brought into A&E or, worse, to the mortuary.

We are legally obliged to educate our children and most elect to send them to school where they expect them to be safe. This mass killing could not have been predicted. The procurator fiscal for the area was informed of the fatalities, and the Edinburgh department of forensic medicine was contacted. We were all ready to respond and deal with this as quickly as we could. Professor Tony Busuttil advised that there would be no benefit in full autopsies on the children: their cause of death was self-evident, and this was agreed. The perpetrator was a local man, Thomas Hamilton. There was much speculation about the reasons for his actions, but we will never know.

As a result of this tragedy there was much lobbying for tighter gun laws and increased security in schools. It took a little time but new laws restricting ownership of guns are in place, and schools are much more secure. In the UK, the safety of the vulnerable outweighs the Americans' right to arms. Aren't all children precious and deserving of a safe environment?

My abiding memory of Dunblane was of driving through eerily silent streets lined with floral tributes, cascading from the pavements onto the road, on my way to the funeral of one of the children. I had never witnessed such a visual example of solidarity in grief to that extent before.

7

Murder Most Foul

'THOU SHALT NOT KILL.' A seemingly simple instruction, literally written in stone, but one that many do not heed. The UK and Ireland are relatively safe places to live, being far down the murder league tables compared to the rest of Europe; the murder rate in the USA is five times our average, while some countries, like El Salvador and Jamaica, are around sixty times our rate of around one murder per 100,000 population. In addition, there are very few random killings in the UK and Ireland: the people you should fear most are your family and 'friends'. Women, the elderly and the young are the most vulnerable in our society.

Mary Whelan was not long married to her husband. On the surface their relationship seemed fine, or as good as most. But while Mary may have been relatively happy, her husband wasn't. Mary was brought into hospital after a suspected fall downstairs. It was alleged that her husband had found her at the bottom of the stairs when he returned home. He phoned the emergency services and attempted CPR as he awaited assistance. The medical staff in the hospital noted marks on her neck while they were treating her. Unfortunately, Mary did not survive. The gardaí were informed that her injuries did not fit with a fall downstairs.

Back at the mortuary it didn't take me long to agree with the medical staff. There was a ligature mark on her neck and small pinpoint haemorrhages around and in her eyes. Without lifting a scalpel, I was of the firm opinion that she had been strangled. There were few other marks on her body, certainly not the pattern of injuries I would have expected if she had fallen downstairs. A careful dissection of her neck confirmed that pressure had been applied, obstructing her windpipe and depriving her of oxygen, for sufficient time to cause her death. This was no fall downstairs. There were grazes, which could have been caused if she had slid on the stairs or had been dragged down. But there was no evidence of injuries to support a fall and, most importantly, no other injuries that could have caused her death. She was healthy. Time would tell if she had been drunk or drugged.

My findings came as no surprise to the gardaí investigating the death. We had two conflicting accounts, mine and Colin Whelan's. I had no doubt about my findings, but was it possible that she had accidentally strangled herself as she fell downstairs, something around her neck getting caught and choking her? Always keep an open mind. Sometimes people have unwittingly altered a scene. In a panic, suddenly faced with someone known to them collapsed and unresponsive, they may move something, even the person, but not remember the exact details when questioned later. So might something have been around Mary's neck that was cast aside or dropped when she was being moved? And was there something that a potential ligature could have caught on? The only thing to do was to return to the scene of the alleged crime. A busload of forensic experts, plus the usual suspects, including the crime-scene manager, a photographer, fingerprinter, ballistics expert, mapper and forensic scientist, went on a day trip to Balbriggan.

The house was neat and tidy. I was shown where the paramedics had treated Mary, in the hall at the bottom of the stairs. There was nothing untoward in the hall. Mary had been wrapped in a duvet when the paramedics arrived: could she have had it wrapped around her, tripped on the stairs, and some part of it had got caught around her neck? The stairs were rather narrow, as expected in modern houses of that era, and we ascended, scrutinising the walls for evidence of scuffing or other damage caused as a person came tumbling down. Upstairs we entered the master bedroom. I was looking for something that could have been used as a ligature. There had been nothing obvious in the hall or on the stairs, and there was nothing lying around the bedroom.

A dressing-gown was hanging on a hook on the door; in my experience, the belts from dressing-gowns are commonly used as ligatures in domestic murders. On first appearances the belt was where it should be, through the loops at the waist of the gown. However, there was red staining of the material at the 'back': could this be blood? I was certain that the belt could have been used as a ligature but, if so, it would have to have been deliberately replaced after she had been strangled.

Not an accident, then? Were we looking at the murder weapon? The belt was taken as evidence and sent to the forensic science laboratory to confirm the staining as Mary's blood. There were also some minute traces of blood in the bedroom, which also needed to be analysed. I was now convinced that there was no other possible explanation other than death due to deliberate ligature strangulation, in the bedroom, with the belt from the dressing-gown.

My work was done, but the investigation was only beginning. She had been murdered, but why and by whom? The staging of the scene turned the spotlight on her husband. Had Colin tried to be too clever? The scenario that unfolded was like something out of fiction. The protagonist, Colin, had increased the amount of life insurance payable on their deaths prior to his marriage to Mary. He was a computer analyst and his computer at work was interrogated. Despite wiping his 'history', it was still possible to follow his browsing history: he had an unhealthy interest in asphyxiation and strangulation. A few weeks after her death, Colin was charged with murdering his wife. Great detective work.

Months before his trial Colin's car was found

abandoned at Howth Head. Had it all been too much and, driven by remorse, he had taken his own life? No, this 'fine' man had staged his suicide, fled the country and reinvented himself, new identity and all. He was hiding in plain sight in a bar in Mallorca. As luck would have it, of all the bars in Mallorca, an Irish woman on holiday popped in and recognised him. His luck had run out. He was extradited back to Ireland and this time made it to trial. He was found guilty of the murder of his wife. His downfall was his greed.

When a colleague announced to the professor in the histopathology department that she was considering forensic pathology as her next career move, he was shocked and said, 'But it's all sex, drugs and violence.' Add in a lust for money and that's forensic pathology in a nutshell.

Only a couple of years later, and only a few miles away in north County Dublin, a woman was found dead. The scene was described as a veritable bloodbath, far removed from the relatively serene scene of Mary Whelan's death, which, in fact, belied the horror of her last few minutes. Rachel O'Reilly's battered and bruised body was found when her mother went to Rachel's house to see why she hadn't turned up for the school run that afternoon.

It was October, and by the time I arrived at the house in the Naul it was dark. I waited outside until the photographer had taken the internal photographs and the Technical Bureau were satisfied that there was a clear path through the house to the body. Preservation of evidence is paramount. This was a difficult scene to navigate – the kitchen, in particular, was awash with blood. Analyses of the bloodstaining may be relevant to determining the circumstances surrounding the death and also the movements of the killer through the scene. It is up to the forensic team to ensure that this is not unnecessarily disturbed, no mean feat when having to hover above the blood, stepping from metal plate to metal plate, then having to balance on a metal plate while examining the body. The living areas were in complete disarray, furniture overturned, drawers pulled out. To my untrained eye it looked as if someone had been searching for something. I could see why this was initially being treated as a burglary that had been disturbed.

Even if it was, Rachel did not deserve such a horrific death. She had been struck with a heavy object several times with some force. There was no finesse to this killing: it was a brutal assault on a young woman. I left, perplexed as to why such violence had been necessary.

The next morning we reconvened in the mortuary for the postmortem examination. This confirmed that she had died from severe head injuries. She had tried to defend herself against the vicious attack. If this was a bungled burglary, why was it necessary to use such excessive force? I am always suspicious when there is evidence of 'overkill' when a woman is murdered. It feels deliberate. It smacks of rage specifically directed towards that person. Would you feel such a depth of emotion towards a stranger? I am not a detective, and I am not a profiler, but over the years I have dealt with many women dying after being brutally beaten or the victim of a knife assault, the wounds running into tens, twenties and more, and their killer is the one who purports to love them, the husband, boyfriend or partner.

I was not surprised to see Rachel's husband, Joe, on *The Late Late Show* pleading for information to help catch her killer. Such public displays always make me suspicious. In my experience relatives are usually stunned and sometimes disbelieving, with a need to see for themselves. Emotions tend to be contained, at least in public. I don't know what goes on behind closed doors. Silent tears are all that is usually seen by the outside world. Maybe it is just the cynic in me that makes me wonder about such an orchestrated display of grief. But I'm not always right, and it is not up to me to identify the murderer. But!

The garda evidence against Joe O'Reilly began to pile up. Advances in technology allowed tracking of his movements on the day of Rachel's death and this did not tally with his accounts of where he said he had been. Messages were also present to another woman. The amount of work in such a technical investigation is phenomenal. The staging of the scene came under scrutiny: if this was a robbery, and the house looked as if it had been pulled apart, why was so little missing and why were some 'stolen' items found in a ditch close to the house? Eventually the gardaí and the DPP felt there was sufficient evidence to charge him with Rachel's murder. Despite his continued protestations of innocence, a jury found him guilty. Poor Rachel – was she just in the way of a new romance? Is murder preferable to divorce? What a twisted world we live in.

But spouse homicide is not restricted to men killing their partners or wives: women are capable of killing. Not long after arriving to take up his post in Glasgow the new professor of forensic medicine went out to the scene of a man stabbed to death. When asked about the case, he described the multiple stab wounds. 'One thing for sure, a woman did not kill this man.'

Our collective reply to this statement? 'Welcome to Glasgow!' The women in England were clearly gentler than a Glasgow woman scorned. Women have been known to snap, usually after years of abuse at the hands of their partner, and in some circumstances can be as violent as any man, after years of pent-up rage. No excuse but, to me, understandable. There is no option for these women. Once it gets to that stage, if they restrain themselves and the man makes a full recovery, the woman can only imagine the repercussions. What will be their punishment for attempted murder, if a late dinner warrants a black eye or a bloody nose?

If we accept that women can be violent and can physically abuse their partners in the heat of the moment, we also have to acknowledge that they can murder in cold blood. A man may plan the murder of his partner, the perceived impediment to a better life, and so too, on occasion, a woman may see her partner as a problem to be disposed of. The difference is that they may coerce their new love interest to deal with the situation, the woman keeping her hands clean.

In 2000 when Gerry McGinley's wife reported him missing probably few in Northern Ireland were worried about the disappearance of this rather unsavoury character. About a year later, a schoolgirl and her family walking in a wooded area across the border in County Leitrim came across a partly buried body. By the time I had trekked up to the scene, the news had sparked speculation that this could be Gerry McGinley. An investigation was launched on both sides of the border in anticipation. The body was found in a shallow grave, naked and wrapped in plastic. It was badly decomposed and therefore identification would be a problem. I was offered the services of a forensic anthropologist from Queen's University to assist. I was delighted: at that time I had yet to find a forensic anthropologist south of the border. Jack Harbison preferred to use a medical anatomist for these purposes, whereas I had worked with forensic anthropologists in Glasgow and abroad and knew the value they added to these investigations. Laureen Buckley proved a valuable asset to the Office of the State Pathologist.

However, it matters not to me who the person is: my role is to identify the cause of death and supply any information that will assist in identification of person, time or place of death. A naked man in a shallow grave is a clear indication that this was not a straightforward death: the presence of blows to the head, causing death, confirmed that this was a murder. The state of the body was in keeping with a time frame of several months. The grave was not where he had been killed: he had been wrapped and transported there after death. The place where he had been killed would have been bloody: even with a clear-up, it is difficult to eradicate all traces of blood.

Using a variety of methods, the identity of the body was confirmed as that of Gerry McGinley. The number one suspect was, of course, his wife, and the new man in her life. As in the case of Mary Whelan, it transpired that Julie McGinley had taken out a large insurance policy against the life of her husband before he 'disappeared'. The Northern Ireland police continued the investigation, and soon the wife and her lover stood trial. They were found guilty of murder.

On the day of the terror attacks on the World Trade Center in 2001, I was on my way to Galway.

An elderly woman had been found dead in her home. She had suffered injuries to her head. I was listening to the radio on my way there when I heard a news flash: a plane had flown into one of the Twin Towers. Shortly afterwards there was an update: another plane, another tower. Like dominoes, the world as we knew it was tumbling down.

My phone rang. My contacts from the UN war crimes work were already getting ready, should their services be required. One of our group was a forensic pathologist from New York, Yvonne Milewski. She had been in touch with Robert McNeil: would our 'gang' be prepared to fly out and help? There were no dissenters. This could be a mammoth task. None of us was able to predict how extensive and difficult it would be. I contacted my boss, Jack Harbison, then the Department of Justice, to seek permission to travel, if need be. They agreed, but the need never arose. Yvonne kept us up to date over the coming days.

Her department was not swamped with bodies in the conventional manner: many were never found and most were blasted to smithereens. The reality was that this became the biggest jigsaw in history, trying to piece together thousands of bodies. The families would have a long wait. The anthropologists were the principal players and today they are still dealing with tiny pieces of tissue and bone being found in and around the site of the Twin Towers. Standing on it is sobering. So many lives lost, so many families devastated. The forensic community is relatively small, but we are all more than willing to lend a hand when necessary.

Meanwhile I had arrived at the scene in Galway. We had gathered to investigate the death of an elderly woman, but we were mindful of what was unfolding just across that expanse of water, the Atlantic Ocean. No matter the scale of the deaths in New York, our duty was to make sure this woman's death was given all our care and attention.

The cottage of the scene was small and unsophisticated. The kitchen-cum-living room was in disarray. An elderly woman lay in a heap on the floor, blood puddled around her head. It was a sorry sight. She had an injury to her head and beside her on the floor was the weapon: the broken-off leg of a kitchen chair. We didn't have to look too far for the culprit: her son.

Every few years a tragedy of this sort occurs,

parents killed by their offspring – the son in the cases I have dealt with, the Sleator family in 2007 and the Cuddihy family in 2014. In both cases the mother and father were older and the families were not physically close to neighbours. The Sleators were shot by their son, who then took his own life. The gun was legally held and at hand. The Cuddihys were killed with an axe, again a tool readily available. Julian Cuddihy stood trial but was found 'not guilty by reason of insanity'; Patrick Sleator was obviously not of sound mind at the time of the deaths. Whatever the catalyst that provokes these attacks, they tend to be violent.

There is much discussion regarding mental health issues and suicide. Families find that difficult to understand, but how can any of us make sense of this when we have never been in their shoes? We like life to be neat and ordered, but it is not. We like to have a reason for actions, but there is not always a defined reason. Life is complex, and so is death.

The shock we feel at someone taking their own life, or killing a spouse or parent, is nothing compared to a parent killing their child. We are programmed to look after our young. Dealing with child deaths is probably the most challenging aspect of my job. I had never had to deal with the death of a child in my immediate family, and even during my medical training, the students were shielded from the harsh reality that at times we cannot prevent death, no matter our medical or surgical expertise. Perhaps I was just blinkered, wanting to believe that I could make a difference, make the sick healthy. Even as a trainee pathologist, unless you had worked in a maternity or paediatric hospital, you might have been aware that certain diseases, cancers and genetic abnormalities caused death in children but you didn't have to face the reality.

Until the day I went to Yorkhill, the paediatric hospital in Glasgow, for the three months required in paediatric pathology to complete my training, in preparation for the exit exam, the second part of the Royal College of Pathology examination. Until that point, child deaths were ethereal – tragic and heartrending, but confined to the pages of a textbook. The routine in the department was postmortems in the morning, 'surgicals' in the afternoon. 'Surgicals' referred to the small pieces of tissue removed during surgery for diagnostic or therapeutic purposes. I was now three years into my apprenticeship, a competent histopathologist, with a special interest in autopsies. The world of forensic pathology was not even on my horizon that first day in paediatric pathology. But it might have been then that a tiny seed was sown.

This was an alien world, partly because everything had shrunk: it was a little like going into a primary school as an adult and realising the chairs and desks are tiny when once they had seemed so big and imposing. The initial shock was seeing little bodies on the mortuary table when I was used to dealing with adults, most of whom had managed to reach a reasonable age. Those little things had either never seen the light of day or never seen it outside a hospital. But I was there to learn, so I swallowed hard and got on with it. It could have been heartbreaking, dealing with miscarriages, stillbirths, a baby with congenital defects that either had had no hope of survival or had died during corrective surgery. But it was there that I witnessed first-hand the strength and courage of the bereaved, and realised that my job was not to mourn with them but to try to provide the answers to their questions. Why did he die? Why wasn't the surgery successful? Was it my fault? Could this happen to another child? Should I have any more children?

Only once did I let my mask of professionalism slip, the day I walked into the little chapel area where the parents were waiting to do the required identification. As I tell my students, when you are meeting the bereaved, remember that they are looking at you, the doctor, to take charge of the situation; you are there to help them. The information I had been given was that this was a sudden death, most likely a 'cot death', the terminology of the time. What I had failed to notice when I had checked the ID form was that there were in fact two forms. I opened the door ready to greet and console the grieving parents but instead of one little Moses basket there were two. Two identical babies, in two identical baskets; postmortems would show that these were cot deaths. I was totally unprepared for this. My mask crumpled and so did I. In contrast to the stoic parents, the doctor was a snivelling wreck.

Luckily the 'real' paediatric pathologist, Professor Angus Gibson, had the good sense to check up on his trainee. I was quickly ushered out. Quite rightly, he told me I was not helping the situation. That was an important lesson for me to learn. It also made me realise that, when dealing with child deaths, make sure that everyone is coping. Sometimes you have to be the responsible adult.

I learned so much in those three months. Little did I know that the relationships I made with the paediatric pathologists would stand me in good stead when I became a forensic pathologist. The realisation that I could cope with child deaths has stood me in good stead throughout my forensic career, and very little reduces me to tears in the mortuary. Apart from the time I sliced into my hand during a postmortem. I hadn't noticed the technician swapping the disposable 'brain' knife for a new blade as I turned to weigh a kidney. I picked up the second kidney and, holding it in my left hand, sliced through to examine the internal structures. The razor-sharp blade sliced cleanly through the kidney and my hand. That brought tears to my eyes. It was also the only time I injured myself, despite dealing with sharp blades for thirty-odd years.

Distancing yourself from the emotions of dealing with death is part of the coping strategy. Only once did it fail me. The emergency services had been called to a flat after a child had collapsed at 'home'. They found the battered body of an infant. This wasn't the first I had dealt with. We now use non-inflammatory terminology, such as 'non-accidental injury' or 'abusive head trauma', but that child had been battered to death. I went to the flat to see the child in situ. The police hadn't sugar-coated it. It was going to be an ordeal. They met me at the close mouth and I followed them into the flat. This was bedsit land, a haven for drug addicts and those living on the verges of society. The smell was appalling, the furnishings sparse and shabby and the detritus of daily surviving, not living, scattered on the floor and any available surface. Utter squalor.

We went through the 'living' quarters and into the 'bedroom'. It was small. There were dirty clothes on the floor. I was careful where I walked. The police in front of me came to a halt, then moved to my side to afford me a clear view of the body. A scrap of a child lay among soiled and crumpled 'bedding', most likely towels, scraps of material and discarded clothes. A child, a little girl, had been abused, tossed aside and left to die. There was only one word fitting to sum up this sight: 'bastards'. But it is not for me to condemn and judge, but to scoop up the little mite and get her out of that hell-hole. She was bruised from head to toe.

There was a stillness in the room, unusual at a scene as there are normally the sounds of chatter, greetings, introductions being made and instructions given. This claustrophobic silence is only 'heard' when dealing with the suspicious deaths of children. I broke the silence by asking for the child's name and details for my notes. 'Samantha O'Brien. She's about two years old. We haven't got her date of birth yet.' I had left my daughter that morning in the care of my sister-in-law, Frances. My daughter is Sarah O'Brien, and then she was just over two. Too close for comfort. But it only spurred me on to make sure that I did the best I could for Samantha. She would never have the opportunity to grow up to become a beautiful, intelligent young woman, but my daughter would.

A few months into my training as a forensic pathologist in Glasgow I came across my first filicide-suicide, or 'family wipe-out', case: a mother had suffocated her sons and taken an overdose. Tiny children lying on mortuary tables designed with adults in mind. The only saving grace: there was no evidence that the mother had abused her children in any way. She had been at the end of her tether.

Twenty years later I encountered a similar scenario with the Grace family. Sharon Grace was separated from the father of her children, Mikahla and Abby. No one knows exactly what problems and issues she was facing, but we do know that on a Saturday night in 2005 she looked for help. With her children in tow, Mikahla, aged four, and Abby, three, Sharon went to the local hospital and asked to see a social worker. There was no out-of-hours service and she was told to return on the Monday morning.

On Sunday morning three bodies were removed from the water at Kaats Strand in Wexford. All three had drowned. But this was no accident: Sharon had walked into the water with her children. She hadn't drugged them or knocked them unconscious, she'd simply walked into the water with her two young children. What happened that Saturday that was so different from any other day? What tipped her over the edge? We will never know. But we do know that she looked for help and didn't find it. We failed her. We decided that some services are more important than others. How many others reach out in despair and find no help? None of us can imagine being so desperate that the only solution is death; so desperate that you take your children by the hand and deliberately walk into the water, knowing that you will all drown.

Much research has been carried out in the USA on such groups of deaths. There are recurring themes: mental health issues, depression, substance or alcohol abuse, stress, lack of support and economic difficulties. Many people weather such stresses and strains, so why do some people respond by killing their family? Again, we never know for sure what was the trigger. We do know that women tend to be less violent, but not always. Men may be more likely to resort to violent means, but not always.

Gregory Fox killed his wife and two sons. That sentence cannot convey the horror that their home contained. Mother, father and two boys, with a lovely house and a local business. We have only his version of the events of that fateful day in July 2001, which ended with his family dead and him seriously injured. The children were on holiday from school, it should have been a lovely day. But something must have been brewing. Gregory Fox felt his wife was unhappy in their marriage. He thought she might be having an affair. They had been out for a few drinks but when they returned to the house an argument broke out. This changed from verbal to physical and before he knew it his wife was dead. He had slashed her neck with a bottle that had broken when the fight escalated.

Hers was the first body I saw. She was lying on the kitchen floor in a pool of blood. She had a large gash on her neck and the postmortem would show that her jugular vein had been slashed. She had obviously fought back and had also been struck with fists or a blunt object. I was to discover that she had a fractured skull. A sad end to a marriage.

But the horrors lay in their sons' bedrooms. Sometimes being able to reconstruct the scenario from the injuries and blood pattern at the scene is a curse. It was apparent from the position of the boys that each had been asleep in bed when their father came in wielding a knife. They did not die unaware of their father's intended actions – perhaps they were awakened by their parents fighting in the kitchen or woke when their dad barged into their rooms. Both boys had been stabbed multiple times. Like their mother, they had tried to fight back. They had got up but couldn't get away. Each died alone in their room in a frenzied attack. I never use 'frenzy' to describe injuries or an assault but no other word comes near to covering what happened to those three people that night.

Gregory's suicide attempt was unsuccessful and he has to live with the consequences of his actions that night. And he has ample time to do so while serving three life sentences.

That was in sharp contrast to the deaths of John Butler and his two children. John had a history of depression and had received treatment for his condition. In November 2010 he was looking after his two children. He left the house alone and drove to a garage where he filled a can with petrol. He was seen driving erratically. He drove the car into a ditch and it burst into flames. His charred body was eventually recovered from the car. Relatives became concerned about the children and gained entry to the family home, where they found the children dead. The scene was peaceful and serene. This was not a man who had lost control but had lost the will to live in this world. Most likely he had thought his children should not have to live in it either.

Around the same time a mother, her two young children and her friend were found stabbed to death in their home. Another disturbing scene. But in this case Sarah Hines was the target, her children and friend merely the fallout. A callous act of viciousness against an ex-partner. There was no regard for the collateral damage, the deaths of 'innocents', the unintended victims.

We must never assume we know or understand the motives behind the deaths of whole families or what complex emotions were involved. If only we could recognise danger signs beforehand . . .

Sometimes the danger lurking in the home is not your family but someone you have invited in, a friend. 'Not guilty by reason of insanity': the verdict came as no surprise to anyone who had followed the trial and heard the evidence. Saverio Bellante had admitted the killing and a whole lot more.

Tom O'Gorman had befriended Saverio, who had become his lodger. They were both intelligent young men and shared a love of chess. No one could have guessed that a game of chess would end as it did. The gardaí were called to the house by Saverio, who said he had killed Tom and eaten his heart. Tom was the devil and he, Saverio, was Jesus Christ and the only way to be rid of the devil was to eat his heart. The gardaí were sceptical and thought that Saverio was laying the ground for a plea of insanity: no one in their right mind would come up with such a story.

In my time I have dealt with murders in which bodies have been mutilated and internal organs removed – a young woman's spleen was stuffed into her mouth and a middle-aged man's penis was shoved down the back of his throat.

I entered the house with an open mind. I have learned over the years not to speculate and wait until I have had a look. There was no doubt that Tom O'Gorman had been brutally murdered: he had been struck on the head with such force that the left side of his skull was shattered and his brain pulverised. There were also knife wounds on his head, neck and chest, as well as on his arms, indicating that he was likely attacked by someone wielding a knife and was struck on the head when he collapsed to the floor. A short, but extremely violent assault.

A dumbbell and a knife lay close to the body and I was of the opinion that, from the appearance of the injuries, those were the weapons used. An unusual finding was a fist-sized hole in the front of Tom's chest. I could see the organs inside his chest and was pretty sure his heart was still in situ. Was the alleged removal of the heart a ruse? Was this in fact a sane and intelligent man who, as the gardaí suspected, was misleading us into thinking he was insane?

Once I had examined the body I went into the kitchen. There was a plate on the table with the remains of a meal and a pan on the stove with some cooked meat in it. It didn't look like heart muscle. The gardaí found a plastic bag in the bin, which contained fresh meat. It looked like lung tissue. I re-examined the cooked 'meat' in the pan and on the plate: it could have been cooked lung tissue. It would be wise to get a psychiatric opinion on Saverio's state of mind.

The postmortem examination confirmed the extent of the external injuries and that part of the right lung had been hacked off. The right lung comprises three lobes, or parts, and two were missing. I examined the cooked tissues and the fresh tissue from the kitchen under the microscope and this confirmed they were lung tissue. But some was missing.

Saverio was diagnosed as schizophrenic by forensic psychiatrists; I am not decrying their expertise in such matters, but all of us in that courtroom had no doubt there was something far wrong with him. This begs the same old questions: how do we keep people safe? How do we spot the signs that someone is struggling or on the brink of a violent outburst? When does 'just a bit odd' become a psychiatric illness?

It's the same old answer: who knows? Mercifully there are relatively few killings of this type. Hard statistics are difficult to come by. I would have liked to compare and contrast the postmortem findings in murders where the verdict was not guilty by reason of insanity with those committed by the 'sane'. Could that research help decide in the early stages if the killer was mad, bad or other? This is not an attempt at profiling. Few murders are committed by the mad and bad, thankfully. The majority are committed by people who lost control, got involved with the 'wrong' crowd, were reckless or simply stupid. The majority did not set out to kill someone. I can sometimes see how a murder happened, but most of us stop short and don't cross that threshold.

Liu Qing and Feng Yue were Chinese students living in Dublin city centre. They had been home to China for the holidays but had returned for the start of term. The emergency services were called to a fire in the flat they had been renting and two bodies were found in the bedroom, lying side by side in the bed, as if they had slept through the blaze. That was immediately suspicious. Despite the stench of burned materials there was the definite odour of accelerant, probably petrol. Now it was looking like an arson attack.

Meanwhile I was a bit worried. Maybe I was overreacting but the bodies were too precise, lying side by side, and they were not dressed for bed, although they might have been taking an afternoon nap when the fire was started, but there was the burnt remains of a strip of material around the young man's neck. We had to get them out and up to the mortuary for postmortem to be sure that they had died in the fire. Another issue was identifying the bodies: we knew who should have been living in the flat but the families of Liu and Feng were in China: someone at college who knew them would have to confirm that the bodies were the two Chinese nationals. A close friend, Yu Jie, was asked to attend at the mortuary. An interpreter was found and we explained the identification procedure to Yu through the interpreter. He nodded his assent.

The city mortuary in Dublin was housed in a Portakabin in the grounds of the fire brigade training centre. It was fitted out as befits a modern mortuary, but space was limited. Family were brought to the back of the building and into the ID room. This was fitted out in a manner that was hoped to be calming for the relatives and respectful to the deceased, but there was no barrier: the families came face to face with their loved ones. This was difficult and traumatic to some, particularly if the death had been violent. Others were grateful for the opportunity to be able to see and even touch their loved ones.

Yu Jie was brought into the room where his friends were lying on trolleys, covered with a sheet. The faces were revealed one by one. This had an instant and dramatic effect on the young student. He collapsed, screaming and wailing. He was obviously traumatised by the ordeal. I was in the next room and was concerned for his welfare, annoyed that the gardaí had been so insensitive, expecting a young man, unfamiliar with our language, country and customs, to be put in such a situation. Little did I know. We tried to calm him down but he was inconsolable. He was escorted home after it was established that he would not be alone.

The postmortems showed that Liu and Feng had been dead before the fire began. They had not inhaled smoke, there had been no coughing and spluttering as the acrid fumes engulfed the flat. The material I had seen around Feng's neck was indeed a ligature. The fire had not erased the tell-tale signs of murder. My interpretation of the pattern of injuries was that they had been attacked and struggled with the attacker or attackers before being strangled, and once dead were dragged into the bedroom and placed on the bed. If both had been in the flat together there were probably at least two killers. It was now up to the gardaí to do the legwork and try to map out the movements of this young couple between their return to Ireland and their deaths.

The one name that kept cropping up was Yu Jie's. CCTV footage from cameras in the area of the flat identified him and Feng together in the vicinity prior to the flat fire, and also Yu on his own close to the flat. The gardaí knew he had money problems and had borrowed from other students. He was brought in for questioning. He confessed to killing his friends because he had heard they had been given money and he intended to get hold of it. He had acted alone, killing Feng first, then waiting until Liu came home and killing her. He dragged them onto the bed, doused the flat in petrol and set it alight. Imagine his horror when he was asked to identify them. His attempts to conceal his crime had failed and he was made to face his victims. He must have thought this was a deliberate ploy by the police – no wonder his reaction in the mortuary was so extreme.

Attempts to conceal a crime are not uncommon, and in Ireland this includes hiding the bodies of murder victims. The difficulty for the gardaí is determining whether or not the deceased was killed where the body was found or thereabouts. Was the victim lured to this remote spot and killed there or the body transported there after they had been killed? Was this planned or a spur-of-the-moment decision?

The most common reaction to doing something bad is to scarper, distance yourself from the scene of the crime. Murder is no different. The immediate thought is to get away, although some stay put and even phone the emergency services. Most murders are impulsive, not planned: the niggling argument that escalates, the discovery of yet another act of infidelity, the drink- or drug-fuelled bravado. Perhaps the woman subject to a constant drip of emotional, verbal or physical abuse dreams of the day it will stop, but do they think the death of their tormentor is the answer? I don't know. It's a big leap from being a law-abiding citizen to a killer.

Some murders are obviously planned. Gangland 'hits' range from the amateur drive-by shootings to planned killings in which the 'unsuspecting' victim arranges a meeting with dubious characters in an out-of-the-way spot. These bodies will be left in situ, but if they are in a car it seems *de rigueur* to set it alight. And, of course, there are the men who decide to dispose of their partner. While men seem happy enough to meet in a dark wood, women are generally not so keen, unless they are having an affair and this is the only secluded spot for clandestine meetings. Most women will be killed indoors. Some will be left where they fall or a half-hearted attempt will be made to hide the body, in the wardrobe or under the bed, in all cases close to home. Discovery will come sooner or later, usually sooner. Out of sight is not out of mind. Bodies are often found because the neighbours complain about the smell.

Anne Shortall's body was discovered barely concealed in the workshop in the grounds of Roy Webster's house. It was another unfortunate tale of 'love' gone wrong, ending in threats to and the attempted blackmail of Roy by Anne. They met, she was killed by blows to the head but then he had the problem of disposal. He wrapped her cocoon-like, probably to prevent blood leaking in his van rather than to conceal the body, eventually deciding to put it in his workshop part-hidden. His saving grace was a conscience: he confessed to his family.

In some cases the killer may have the foresight to stage the scene, to try to make the death seem incidental to another crime, or even to appear to be a suicide. This usually indicates a degree of planning. However, crime-scene investigators are alert to any discrepancy that may not ring true. A case of knowing something is not quite right, but not sure what is wrong, that there is doubt enough to warrant careful scrutiny of the death. We are ever vigilant and take very seriously any inkling that something does not ring true.

Bodies may be set alight or disposed of in water – rivers, lakes or the sea. Fire and water can be equally destructive but each causes different problems. Fire deaths are always treated as suspect: was this an accidental fire, an arson attack or a means of concealing murder? The majority of house fires are accidental – the dropped cigarette of the sleeping drunk, the electrical fault, the untended candle. Although the house might be almost completely incinerated, there are usually sufficient clues for the fire investigators to identify the source. As soon as there is any suggestion, or whiff, of accelerant used to ignite a fire it is treated as an arson attack. That deals with the cause.

It is for the pathologist to determine whether or not the death of an individual was due to the fire or something else, not necessarily suspicious. The elderly person making dinner and a tea-towel goes up in flames: the shock may be sufficient to cause a heart attack. The postmortem shows they had collapsed and died before the fire took hold: there was no soot in the airways and the heart was old and scarred. The middle-aged man with a cough who had been out drinking the night before: there is some soot in his airways, he has a mild chest infection, his carbon monoxide is raised and his blood alcohol is high. If the cause of the fire is known and appears accidental, it is safe to say that the fire caused death. However, if the fire was due to an arson attack, the postmortem findings will be interpreted differently: soot in the airways and a high carbon monoxide level indicate that this was murder by fire, despite the state of his health and the fact he had been drinking.

Fire scenes are unsafe and therefore pathologists do not usually make house calls, but one morning I was called out to one in Glasgow. It was an affluent area, a beautiful old stone building, high ceilings, period features and full of antiques. Well, it had been, but no more. The fire had raged through the house pretty quickly. The grandfather and his two grandchildren had escaped but for some reason the woman who owned the house, the daughter and mother of the escapees, had not. She was fit and healthy by all accounts and should have been able to get out.

I was given a hard hat and brought into the crumbled shell of the once handsome house. Everything was blackened with soot. The upper floors had caved in and the house had concertinaed, two floors of living compressed into piles of rubble and the remains of furniture. I was there to see the body of the woman *in situ*. It took me several minutes to be able to appreciate the outline of a head and shoulders – everything had the same charred black appearance. The fire-fighters had a plan of the house's layout and, from where her body now was, they were of the opinion she had been in the upstairs bathroom. The body was removed to Glasgow city mortuary for postmortem.

It was badly charred beyond recognition but there was distinctive jewellery on the remains, which was identified by family members. There was soot in her airways and a high level of carbon monoxide in her blood; her death was due to the fire. I could not explain why she had been unable to escape. Was she somehow trapped in the bathroom?

Accelerant was found so this was now a case of arson, and murder by fire. The culprit, the teenage son, eventually confessed to starting the fire in a fit of pique against his mother. No explanation was given as to why she was the only one who didn't manage to escape. The extent of the building's destruction precluded any meaningful interpretation of the scene: the bathroom no longer existed – the door was a pile of ash, its metal fixings unidentifiable. The forensic team does not always hold all the answers.

In contrast to this was the death of a woman in a fire in Cork. Neighbours noted smoke and flames billowing out of the window of Olivia Dunlea's upstairs bedroom. Ordinarily this would have been treated as an accidental death but the investigating officers and the coroner asked if I would visit the scene as the local pathologist, Margot Bolster, was on holiday. By the time I arrived in Cork, having driven down from Dublin, the house had been examined and the team were getting ready to move the body. Downstairs was coated with a layer of soot, but apart from a little fire damage to the kitchen table, nothing of note. The stairwell was similarly smoke-damaged, but as we ascended there was more evidence of heat damage.

Once I reached the top landing I could see the extent of the fire. The door to the front bedroom where Olivia had been sleeping was part burned through. In the bedroom, fire debris covered every surface. The ceiling was almost gone and the loft contents had tumbled down onto the bed, with the barely discernible, burned remains of a body, lying face down. Little could be seen with the body in that position so it was decided to move it to the mortuary for a full examination. We were still assuming that she had been smoking in bed, fallen asleep and set the bedclothes alight.

In the mortuary I set about removing and describing the clothing, then the fire damage to the body. There was a mark on Olivia's neck, which on closer inspection looked like a stab wound. I cleaned the soot from the skin in this area and found a small cluster of stab wounds. My heart sank. This death had gone from accident to homicide in just a few seconds. I turned to the scenes-of-crime crew and told them I had bad news.

No one took much interest: they were all busy sorting out production bags and photographing the remnants of cloth, assuming this was an accidental fire death. 'She's been stabbed.'

Jimmy the photographer stopped what he was doing and came across to me, camera poised. 'She's not kidding.'

The others scurried over. Olivia had been stabbed. She had not caused the fire, which had been set deliberately by her attacker. This was now a homicide investigation, whether the stab wounds or the fire was the cause of her death.

Fast forward to the first trial. I explained my findings: the victim had been stabbed, left for dead, and the fire had been started. Thick smoke was not lining her airways but I had found soot particles in them when I examined her lungs under the microscope. In addition her blood carbon monoxide was raised, not to a lethal level but sufficient for me to opine that she was alive when the fire started. Her ex-boyfriend, Darren Murphy, pleaded guilty to manslaughter but this was rejected by the DPP: he was to stand trial for the murder of Olivia Dunlea. He was found guilty but that verdict was overturned on appeal. At the retrial the jury could not decide between guilty or innocent. At the third trial he was found guilty of murder. Another failed attempt to conceal a homicide.

The main concern when investigating a fire is that this is a smokescreen to hide the true cause of death: a homicide. As a method of concealing homicide, fire is not efficient. Identification and determination of the cause of death of a fire victim has been unsuccessful in very few instances, no matter the extent of the fire damage. Complete incineration of a body requires high temperatures for a fairly long period. Crematoria require bodies to be subject to temperatures of at least 760 degrees centigrade for ninety minutes, or more, to burn off all the water, soft tissues and organs, leaving behind only bone. A wood fire reaches temperatures of around 600 degrees so an accelerant is required to ensure a raging fire that will incinerate a body. Only if a high-temperature fire is left to burn itself out will the body be cremated. Despite her husband's attempt, Dolores McRae was still identified from the remains of the bonfire in Donegal.

When trying to use fire to destroy the evidence

of a homicide, it is a mistake to attempt to set the body alight. On several occasions I have seen newspapers and the like piled up around the body and set on fire. The clothing may catch and there may be some scorching of the body but the evidence remains. One elderly man was strangled by his girlfriend. She panicked and managed to pull his body into the hall so that anyone looking through the front window wouldn't see it. She piled some rubbish around his head, set it alight and made a run for it. The fire soon puttered out and was as cold as he was when a neighbour came looking for him. The mistake the girlfriend had made was not removing the tie she had used to strangle him. It was partly burned but with fragments of the material still around his neck. The postmortem proved he had been strangled and that the fire was an afterthought.

In another case, a young man stabbed the mother of his friend and tried to set her clothing alight. Even if he had been successful in starting a raging fire there was a flaw: not only had she been stabbed multiple times, but the handle of the knife had broken off and the blade was still embedded in her chest.

Bodies recovered from water are strangely more

difficult to deal with than those recovered from fire. The UK and Ireland are wet islands, overflowing with rivers and lakes. Drownings are common: the fisherman lost at sea, the youngsters larking about in the river, with or without alcohol on board, the toddler falling into the pond, and many variations on ill-fortune or stupidity. Drowning is the method of choice in some suicides, some deliberately weighing down their body or tying their wrists together to ensure they cannot 'save' themselves. These are always treated as potential homicides until proven otherwise.

In Glasgow, a city with a river at its heart, water attracted people for fun and for tragedy. This is where I met a man with a most peculiar job. In the late 1700s a Glasgow businessman left money to the Faculty of Surgeons for the rescue and recovery of drowning persons. The Glasgow Humane Society was set up and undertook to reward gallant rescuers. In the late 1800s they appointed a full-time rescuer. That post still exists today. When I started in the forensic medicine department in 1985, George Parsonage was in post, having taken over from his father a few years earlier. He was the keeper of the Clyde and patrolled its waters daily. He was called to recover live and dead bodies from his station. He was still rowing when I was in Glasgow although latterly he upgraded to motor power. He delivered the bodies to the shore, just a short journey from the city mortuary. No matter how or why you went in, George was the man to get you out, alive if possible. The dead were not pleasant to deal with, particularly if the body had been in the water for some days, but he never faltered and he was always available. He is not long retired.

Water is destructive to the body but it still doesn't wash away all traces of a crime. In England there was a series of sex-related homicides and the women's bodies were dumped in water. Despite a lapse of days, and even a few weeks, before the bodies were discovered, traces of sperm were still recoverable. DNA profiles identified the perpetrator.

In Waterford a woman was reported missing by her work colleagues when she failed to turn up, without explanation. The gardaí carried out an extensive investigation into her whereabouts. About two weeks later a body was recovered from the River Suir, in Waterford, which was identified as Meg Walsh. At this stage in the investigation there was little information regarding the circumstances of her death. Could this have been an accident, a suicide or a homicide? I was asked to carry out the postmortem.

Meg had last been seen alive on the 1st of October. I was mindful that a body in a river for a couple of weeks would be showing marked changes, and could also have been damaged by marine life and river traffic. The effects of immersion were such that visual identification was not ideal and there was postmortem damage to her extremities, such as would be expected. There was no doubt that she had suffered severe blunt trauma to her head. That extent of trauma would have been sufficient to render her unconscious and cause her death, but I had to prove that she was alive when struck on the head and that the injuries were not sustained after she had gone into the water.

Her skull was fractured and the pattern of the fractures was more consistent with a blow to the head from a small heavy object than from part of a boat. Generally, peri-mortem injuries can be distinguished from postmortem injuries by the presence of haemorrhage into the tissues around an injury. The splits in her scalp were bloodless, but water gets into open wounds and leaches out any red blood cells in the tissues. So, although I was sure her death was due to a head injury and that her body had been disposed of in the river, I wanted proof.

If she had been murdered there might be other injuries, even defence injuries. Careful dissection of her limbs provided the answer. Although her body showed no obvious injuries, under the skin on the back of her right hand there was a large bruise and one of her hand bones, a metacarpal, was broken: a classic defence injury caused in this case when the hand was struck by a weapon as she tried to protect herself from blows to her head. Just to be sure, there was one further test I could carry out: a diatom test.

Diatoms are little marine insects, invisible to the naked eye, which are essentially harmless. They can be a useful marker for death due to drowning. During the drowning process, water gets into the airways, blocking air from the lungs. Death is due to asphyxia, lack of oxygen to the brain. Meanwhile water is being actively sucked into the lungs as the person panics. The diatoms in that water travel deep into the lungs, then swim into the capillaries in the air sacs and into the general circulation; diatoms will be found in the internal organs, remote from the lungs. In contrast, if a lifeless body is dumped in water, water may swill into and out of the mouth but is not drawn into the lungs, and there is no circulating blood to take any foreign material to the other organs. First, the water has to be tested for the presence of diatoms: there are hundreds, if not thousands, of varieties, and the exact types present must be identified for comparison purposes. Ciaran Driver, the senior biomedical forensic scientist in our department, prepared slides from water samples and tissue samples from the body and screened them for diatoms.

No match was made. Although the test is not 100 per cent fool-proof, it bolstered my opinion that Meg Walsh had been murdered and her body thrown into the water to conceal the crime. Her husband stood trial but was found not guilty; her murder remains unsolved.

In contrast, Patryk Krupa was alive when he was put into the water. Patryk had fallen foul of a group to whom he owed money. He was picked up by a couple of men. His friends could not stop them and had watched helplessly as he was taken away. They were concerned for his safety and reported him missing. His friends joined in the search and found Patryk's body floating in the Shannon. Attempts to resuscitate him were unsuccessful. A full forensic team attended at the scene.

It was obvious to me that he had been badly

beaten about the head. A postmortem would uncover the precise cause of death. The Technical Bureau had examined the shore in the immediate area and brought my attention to 'drag' marks in the pebbles from under a bridge to the edge of the water. Patryk had been dragged there. There was no evidence that he had struggled: was he unconscious or dead before he had gone into the water?

The postmortem confirmed that Patryk had suffered head injuries that would have rendered him unconscious but not caused immediate or rapid death. The shocking finding was that his lungs had the typical waterlogged appearance of death by drowning: an unconscious Patryk had been callously dragged down to the water's edge and left to drown. Two men were found guilty of his murder.

The perfect murder has yet to be discovered. Attempts to conceal the manner of death as something other than homicide are seldom successful. Forensic pathologists and the police are suspicious by nature and are always looking beyond the obvious. Concealing the body may be more successful but that also depends on there being no suspicion that someone has gone missing or that a crime could have been committed against a missing person. Very few can disappear without a trace, no one noticing their absence.

Therefore, to commit the 'perfect murder', one has not only to dispose of the person and their body in such a manner as will not be detected but also to have a plausible explanation for their apparent disappearance. No traces of a murder, no traces of a body and a watertight alibi. Remember Locard's Principle: every contact leaves a trace. It is well-nigh impossible to get all three right. There is always a slip-up. At least in the murders we know about. Even if you wash the blood off your hands, it is almost impossible to get rid of all trace evidence.

A few killers will transport the body to a location other than where the killing took place. Bodies may be taken to remote areas and dumped or buried. Robert Holohan was eleven years old when he disappeared after leaving home on his new BMX bike on 4 January 2005. The last-known sighting was when he visited a neighbour, Wayne O'Donoghue. They were described as good friends even although Wayne was several years older than Robert. When it got dark his mother was concerned and the alarm was raised. His bike was found abandoned at the side of the road.

For eight days friends, neighbours, gardaí and volunteers scoured the local area for Robert. With each passing hour the chances of him being found alive became more remote. Wayne O'Donoghue had taken part in the search. On 12 January he confessed to his father that he had killed Robert and dumped his body in undergrowth in an isolated ditch at Inch Strand. The police found it and contacted me. It was in a location difficult to access and the danger was that vital trace evidence could be lost if too many people disturbed the scene. I was told that the body was wrapped in plastic bags and there was little for me to see, but if I travelled over the next day I could view it in daylight in situ.

Rather than trample the undergrowth, it was decided that a bird's eye view was ample: it was not necessary to be within touching distance of the body. I was sent up in a cherry-picker and hovered over the body at a great height. I needed to appreciate the terrain and the vegetation surrounding it so that I could decide whether any marks on Robert's body could have been caused by being caught on or dragged over the rough undergrowth.

In the mortuary we had to establish our forensic strategy: how best to recover trace evidence. If a body has been wrapped in a material such as plastic, it will hold the imprint of fingerprints, or if the limbs have been bound together with tape, or tape put over the mouth, as in the case of Anne Shortall, we must take care not to smear the prints. The material may be 'printed', then removed, or cut off with care and taken to the laboratory for examination. If a ligature is tied around the neck, wrists or ankles, the area of interest will be the knot, in this case DNA transferred during tying; the ligature will be cut distant from the knot. How the evidence will be harvested is a group decision. Sometimes trace evidence will be taken at the scene if some may be lost in transit, but if the body is in an exposed area or cramped conditions it may be best to remove it to the mortuary and take the evidence there.

With Robert Holohan, access to the body at the scene was difficult and it had to be moved before we could make any decisions. It would have been a long, laborious process to print the wrappings while on the body so I tentatively cut them open and, with the minimum of handling, removed them and handed them over to the finger-printer.

A child was revealed and now it was for all of us present to try to ascertain what had happened to him.

On first inspection there was little to indicate why he had died. He had not been subject to any obvious violence – yes, there were bruises but every child will show minor injuries from their normal, active lives. Robert had obviously died suddenly. If it was from some natural disease, I would have assumed any person with him would immediately look for assistance. When Robert died, the person with him hid the body, so the only conclusion was that some action by that person had been responsible for Robert's death. The external findings were subtle, a few marks around the neck and scant tiny pinprick haemorrhages around the eyes. This suggested he could have been asphyxiated. A specialised examination of the internal structures of the neck showed small bruises in the muscles but little else of relevance. A healthy boy appeared to have died after his throat was compressed. A few other investigations needed to be carried out, but this was a homicide.

Wayne admitted that he had had words with Robert, who had thrown pebbles at his car. He had grabbed the boy by the neck but when he let go Robert crumpled to the ground, dead. He had carried him into the house and into the bathroom, where he threw water over Robert's face, to no effect. He wrapped the body in black plastic bags, bundled it into the boot of his car and drove to the remote spot where he had left it.

Wayne was charged with murder. At his trial his account of the events leading to Robert's death was accepted by the judge and jury and he was found not guilty of murder but guilty of manslaughter.

In some cases, more strenuous efforts are made to conceal bodies: they may be spirited away to remote locations, with no connection to either party, and graves dug deep. During the search for the 'Disappeared' in Northern Ireland, I had the good fortune to meet the archaeologist Niamh McCullough. She has the tenacity of a bulldog. I would have found it soul-destroying to spend months searching areas of interest without success. But she soldiered on. Niamh has become the go-to archaeologist as soon as the gardaí have information as to the potential burial site of a murder victim.

The last case I worked with her was that of James Nolan. The story began as many do: in 2011 a man walking his dog on the beach at

Dollymount Strand in Dublin came across an arm. The finding of bones and body parts on beaches is more common than you might think. The majority are animal, but occasionally a human bone pops up. This does not necessarily spark a murder hunt: most bodies in the sea are those of fishermen and the occasional accidental or suicidal drowning. Efforts will always be made to identify the owner of a human bone, but mostly these are futile. If there is flesh on bone our chances are better. 'Hands' and 'arms' are commonly brought to our attention but they usually turn out to be the flipper of some marine mammal.

The body bag arrived in the mortuary and I had a chat with the garda who delivered it to glean what little they knew, which wasn't much. In the postmortem dissection room, I unzipped the bag and immediately Carl Lyon, the technician, and I looked at one another: 'Think we've got a murder on our hands.' The young guard almost choked on his coffee when I told him to get on to his superior officer and send the Technical Bureau down here.

The arm had been carefully, and fairly expertly, severed from the body. I have seen bodies recovered from water that have been damaged by the propeller of a boat. This was the precise action of a sharp implement, not the hacking action of a propeller blade. Large areas of skin had been carved out, exposing the underlying muscle, and the fingertips had been deliberately cut off. The damage to the skin and fingers could not be attributed to nibbling crabs and crustaceans: someone had been making sure we did not identify the person whose arm was lying on my postmortem table. Descriptions of tattoos and fingerprints would be on file if this person had had any dealings with the gardaí.

Although this took place before the Irish DNA database was set up, tissues were sent for DNA analysis. A body or body part washing up on a beach in Ireland might not necessarily be Irish or have gone into the water off the coast of Ireland. Bodies go overboard or off the coast of the UK and end up in the water around the Irish coast or in the nets of trawlers. They are not necessarily 'local'. The DNA profile was sent to the UK, just in case.

Bingo! A direct hit. James Nolan had been charged with a relatively minor motoring offence in the UK and his DNA was on the UK DNA database. James Nolan had been seen last in 2010. Had no one missed him?

We all thought that other parts of him were

bound to turn up sooner or later. Time passed and I had almost forgotten about the severed arm. In 2017 I was informed by the gardaí that they had received information on the whereabouts of the rest of James Nolan. While they were investigating a suspect suicide, a letter had come to light. In it, the deceased man had confessed to killing James Nolan. He stated that he had strangled him and had cut the body into pieces, which he had then disposed of in a variety of locations. The arm found in 2011 had apparently been thrown into the Tolka river. Other body parts had been strewn around County Monaghan and some more was allegedly buried in Tolka Valley Park. The gardaí had been searching certain locations in Monaghan, without success, but were about to embark on a dig in the valley park under the direction of the forensic archaeologist, Niamh.

Niamh had a wealth of experience under her belt at surveying territory, looking for evidence that the terrain had been altered in the past and using specialised equipment to 'see' underground. By the time I arrived on the scene she had excavated the most likely site where a body could be buried, deep in undergrowth on a steep embankment. I was glad I had swapped heels for wellington boots. I watched as, layer by layer, vegetation and soil were scraped away under her eagle eye, the Technical Bureau doing the heavy lifting. Suddenly the outline of a body began to emerge from the earth. We all crowded in as Niamh gingerly brushed aside the loose soil. This was no buried dog or dumped rubbish: it was a torso wrapped in clothing. My instinct was to push Niamh aside, grab a shovel and release the body from its makeshift grave, but I have learned to bide my time: the body would be in my domain within hours and then I could uncover its secrets. As we stood in that little copse, I thought how difficult it must have been to bury that torso and wondered where the rest of James Nolan was. It would take DNA analysis to identify the torso as his. Great pains had been taken to prevent the murder coming to light, but a guilty conscience had won. Thanks to Niamh, we were one step closer to discovering the fate that had befallen James Nolan.

Dismembering a body may seem a practical solution to getting rid of it, but instead of one large piece there are six or more to dispose of, depending on how diligent you are. (If the cuts were cleanly made through a joint it's probable that someone with anatomical knowledge, medical, science, vet or butchery, was responsible.) Next, what do you use? A large knife, an axe or a saw all leave telltale marks on the skin and bone, which can be used to identify the tool. Where do you dismember the body? You need seclusion and space. Do you transport it to another location, which defeats the purpose of dividing it up for ease of getting rid of it, or stay put?

A mistake many have made is to try to dismember a body in a bath: this restricts access to it, but also traces will be left behind. It is a messy business and difficult. Now what? Put the pieces into something, a suitcase or a 'carry-all', or wrap them in plastic, paper or material? And then what? Take a piece at a time or try to dump all the parts at once?

I have seen every permutation of the above and pieces of the body usually surface, even if the killers are not caught. It is not just Locard's Principle you need to be wary of but the doggedness of the gardaí or police.

Burial of a body takes time and a lot of effort and therefore needs to be carried out somewhere secluded. In fact, if people hold their nerve, a body might never be discovered. In Ireland it has long been suspected that six women who went missing in the 1990s were murdered and their bodies concealed. The trail has long grown cold in every case, but they are not forgotten. If their bodies have been buried somewhere in Ireland, their remains would be skeletonised by now. Every bone, body part or body uncovered is treated as the potential discovery of one of these women and the Office of the State Pathologist is informed. If a bone is possibly human, we refer it to the forensic anthropologists.

In two cases of concealed homicide, the bodies were well hidden in their makeshift graves but still they were uncovered. Robert McAuley was murdered in Scotland in 1996 by the father of his partner in a hammer attack and was also strangled. Two friends of the killer were roped into helping dispose of the body, which was wrapped in a carpet and buried in woods near Harthill, twenty miles or so from Glasgow. Unfortunately, one of the friends could not keep the information to himself and told a 'friend', who told the police. Even armed with details of the burial it was no mean feat to find the concealed remains.

Marie Greene went missing on 13 February 2011. She worked as a prostitute in Athlone, and Jimmy Devaney was one of her regulars.

She threatened to expose their relationship to his family, and over a fairly long period he gave her money, presumably buying her silence. She began to demand larger and larger sums. He arranged to meet her to 'discuss' this issue, an argument ensued and Marie was stabbed several times to the head, neck and trunk, and died from a stab wound to her heart. This left Jimmy with a major problem: a dead woman in his van. The rendezvous had been in a remote area outside Athlone, a perfect place to dispose of a body. He drove down a track far from the main road and left the body in a ditch in the bog-land, partly hidden by the undergrowth. He returned to the pub he had been drinking in earlier and it was noted that he was bloodstained and muddy.

The next day, he went back to the scene of his crime and dug out a shallow grave. Marie was covered over and might well have remained unseen for a long time. The gardaí were investigating her disappearance when Jimmy Devaney came to their attention. He was taken in for questioning and eventually disclosed where he had buried her. On 22 February her body was unearthed. Jimmy Devaney was found guilty of the manslaughter of Marie Greene.

Just how many bodies remain undiscovered we will never know. Unless accidentally discovered by the man or woman walking a dog, we have to rely on a pang of conscience. Had Jimmy Devaney not come to the attention of the gardaí, would he have caved in? We'll never know. How many killers are still at large, hoping that a body is never found? Who knows? All the families of missing persons can hope for is that they will turn up safe and well, with stories to tell of their adventures. All dread the knock on the door that heralds the words, 'The body of a young woman has been found and we believe it to be the remains of . . .'

Finding a body in a quiet, secluded out-of-the-way location is not always an indication of an attempt to conceal a death. It may be that the intention was to conceal another crime and the death was incidental. Sexual assaults are covert operations. A solitary victim is targeted and there is a need for privacy; measures are taken to ensure that what is about to happen is unseen. These are often opportunistic assaults and the attacker is not armed or uses a weapon only as a threat: death is incidental to the intention to rape. This contrasts with the intention of serial and sadistic killers where fatal battery is integral to a sexual assault. One must also be mindful of the possibility of accidental death – for example, by suffocation, or from natural causes, usually a heart attack – during clandestine consensual sexual activity.

In one instance a part-naked portly gentleman was found dead on the stairs of an apartment block. His clothing was scattered around him. There were a few scratches and grazes on his body but no obvious cause for his collapse, or state of undress. The police were called. They did not have to look far for the culprit. There was a resident in the block, whose reputation as a comforter to lonely gentlemen was well known to the police. She lived on the next landing up and, when confronted, confessed that the man on the stairs was one of her clients and had collapsed during a rather energetic session. She had panicked and managed to drag him out of her flat and down a flight of stairs. It was rather awkward when his wife attended the mortuary to identify him, although she was neither upset about his death nor the address at which he had met his demise. He was not the first, and certainly won't be the last, person to die during a sexual act.

The investigation of sex-related homicides is challenging for all the forensic experts involved.

Determining the cause of death is relatively straightforward but the difficulty lies in gathering evidence to support a sexual assault having taken place and to identify the perpetrator. There is usually evidence of a struggle, as one would expect if the victim was pounced on unawares, the actual amount of force used to subdue them being relative to their resistance and the discrepancies in height and weight of the two parties.

Sex-related homicide is rare when compared with the number of rapes and other sexual assaults per year. In Ireland about fifteen hundred cases of sexual assault are reported to the gardaí every year, but this is the tip of the iceberg: approximately ten thousand calls are made annually to the rape crisis helpline. There are more female than male victims. The women range mainly from eighteen to fifty years old, and in more than 50 per cent of assaults the perpetrator is known to the victim, ranging from a close relationship, to the guy who offered to buy them a drink in the pub.

Why do some sexual assaults end in death? Is it an escalation from sexual assault to rape to rape-homicide? Is a serial killer just embarking on his career or has he moved jurisdiction to prevent discovery? Or is it just panic?

Sometimes the victim is in the wrong place at the wrong time. Sister Philomena Lyons was one such. She was not the intended victim and perhaps that is why she was killed: the intention was to rape one woman but the perpetrator had to settle for another, an older woman, a nun. Sister Philomena was on her way to a bit of a do when she was attacked in December 2001 in Ballybay, County Monaghan. Her attacker found her alone, waiting for the bus. She was grabbed and dragged from the street to a field behind her convent, hidden from view by a hedge. Later her luggage was found and a search of the local area uncovered her body.

It was obvious from the position of her body and the state of her clothing that she had been sexually assaulted. The postmortem showed that she had been strangled with her scarf. This is not unusual: manual or ligature strangulation is a common cause of death in these circumstances. The original intention had not been to kill, and often the lack of injuries elsewhere on the body confirms that the attacker was unarmed. The ligature may be left in place or there may be bruises or scratches on the neck, caused when it is grabbed and squeezed, the resulting petechial pinpoint haemorrhages in the eyes and on the face confirming this as the cause of death. Death is not immediate, but unconsciousness is, and as it descends, struggling ceases. Mercifully the sexual assault occurs while the victim is in this comatose state. While using clothing as a ligature is common in these attacks, bricks or rocks lying on the ground might also be used to subdue the victim – which unfortunately can also cause death.

Rape-homicides are the extreme end of the spectrum of sexual assaults and show life-threatening injuries, but in non-fatal sexual assaults up to 45 per cent will show some injuries. These range from relatively minor to some requiring medical attention. There may be injuries to the mouth due to a blow or a hand clamped over it, there may be a mix of bruises, grazes and lacerations caused in a struggle, during attempts to restrain or by punches or kicks, as well as bites and marks caused by bindings or restraints. Bites are associated with such assaults and are rich sources of forensic evidence, identification of the biter made possible through their dentition and DNA.

The next step is to collect evidence to support an allegation of a sexual assault. First, the examiner, a forensic physician or a forensic pathologist, depending on whether the victim has survived or died, will look for the specific injuries caused during sexual acts. While this is an important part of differentiating an assault from a sexual assault, the examiner must be open-minded. Research has shown that injuries are caused during consensual sexual intercourse about 50 per cent of the time, usually no more than a bit of chafing, but bruising and bleeding can occur. Finding sex-specific injuries does not corroborate a complaint of rape. Conversely, the majority of sexual assaults are on women who are sexually active adults, many of whom will have had children, and there may be no sex-specific injuries. We have to be aware that their absence does not exclude rape and their presence does not confirm it. After an examination we can state only that there was or was not evidence of an assault and that there was or was not evidence of a sexual act. The doctor does not make the diagnosis of rape. Having said that, in the extreme cases of injury, and death is extreme, you could be forgiven for stating that this was more likely a non-consensual sexual act, a rape.

Sister Philomena had been sexually assaulted, but the next step was to gather the evidence to identify her attacker. Her clothing and belongings were taken, the clothing to be examined for stains, body fluids, hairs and fibres, her glasses to be examined for fingerprints. The body was pored over for any hairs, fibres or dried fluid. Her fingernails were examined: one was broken and a hair was caught in it. Swabs were sent to the forensic science laboratory to examine for sperm and, if possible, get a DNA profile of the attacker. I took standard samples from her for comparison with anything found, for elimination purposes. That was the physical evidence covered.

Meanwhile the gardaí were questioning everyone in the vicinity and trying to locate anyone who cropped up on local CCTV footage on the morning Sister Philomena was attacked. Every man was asked to give his fingerprints and a DNA sample for 'elimination' purposes.

All fell into place: the assailant was caught on CCTV on the street at about the time of the attack; his fingerprint, taken voluntarily, matched a print on Sister Philomena's glasses, and his DNA was a match for DNA lifted from her clothing. He was asked to supply the clothing he had been wearing, which matched fibres found on Sister Philomena's. Edmond Locard would have been delighted.

Another sad case was one of opportunism. A girl

was raped and murdered in Galway in 2007, just three days after she arrived in Ireland. A local man walking home noticed a rucksack and purse on the ground, then something pale in undergrowth. What he did not expect to find was the body of a young woman. It was hidden from public view but she had been pulled off the pathway into the bushes where the assault took place. There was no attempt to ensure she wasn't found – her killer was unconcerned, such was his arrogance. Perhaps he should have been a little less careless.

As always, the forensic team travelled down from Dublin Garda HQ and I came from Swords. The purse contained an ID card so the gardaí had a potential identity: a Swiss student, Manuela Riedo, seventeen years old. In single file we walked in her footsteps along the route she must have taken as she followed the shortcut from her host home in Renmore to meet up with fellow students in Galway city centre. Close to where the body lay, the path was taped off and we made a detour through the rough, overgrown vegetation. In a natural hollow lay the body of a young woman, partly covered by a coat held down by large rocks. There was no doubt that she had been beaten, strangled and sexually assaulted. Her clothing was strewn around her.

There was a subdued air as we all busied ourselves, automatically switching into professional mode.

We all have our roles, and we all recognise our limitations. This case was going to hinge on the forensic evidence so a forensic scientist was required at the scene, now. I knew what I was dealing with, a young woman raped and killed – the postmortem would confirm only the finer points – but I was not going to risk losing one vital cell clinging to her body that might identify her killer: I would remain hands-off for the moment. While we waited, we had a look around. This was obviously a little hidey-hole used by illicit drinkers and drug-takers, as well as a secluded spot for 'romantic' liaisons, inferred from the detritus left behind by the visitors. I was not surprised to be shown a condom wrapper and condoms hanging from the branches of a nearby tree and discarded beer cans. Every artefact was photographed in situ, bagged and labelled. The pile of evidence was growing into a sizeable mound. No one knows at this stage of an investigation what will be relevant.

By now we had our 'forensic' version of the circumstances. The gardaí would make further investigations and collate the evidence to prepare their version. But the killer was out there somewhere, and he would have his version of what had happened. At the centre of this investigation was Manuela, and our hope was to do her justice. We stood around her, as if we could shield her from more harm, forming a closed circle. Each of us was directly linked to her, each forensic expert and investigator abutting the next but never stepping into the space of their neighbour. The circle around her grew with each step of the investigation, from scene to court, as the family, friends, witnesses, the DPP, the judge and the jury joined it, all looking inwards towards Manuela.

At the scene I made way for the forensic scientist to join the circle and knelt at Manuela's side to help him if required. The usual trace evidence would be taken – hair, fingernail scrapings, swabs from the mouth, vagina, anus, neck, wrists, ankles and breasts; this evidence is more usually gathered by the pathologist. The forensic scientist more commonly attends the scene when their expertise and advice are needed in more unusual cases.

Mercifully, probable stranger rape-homicides are rare, and all our expertise was warranted from the early stages so nothing was overlooked or missed completely. A technique used by forensic scientists in these cases is known as body mapping. It involves covering the body with small pieces of tape, a centimetre or so square, much like the scales of a fish. Every part of the body is covered, every piece of tape numbered, like a giant jigsaw. The pieces of tape will be processed and DNA profiles obtained. The hope is that the scientist will be able to produce a map of the parts of the body touched by the attacker: neck grabbed, wrists gripped, breasts touched, pulled by the ankles. It is laborious and painstaking, and requires complete concentration. A silent crowd watched as he worked.

Eventually, the circle broke and the body was carried back to Renmore, then taken to the mortuary to complete the examination. The only difficulty I had was that I could not give an accurate time of death. The gardaí had a rough idea of when Manuela had left the host family home but nothing else until her body was found the next evening. The only possibility was to bring in another 'ologist.

Professor Patricia Wiltshire is an expert in the field of forensic palynology, ecology and all things botanical. Could she analyse the stomach contents and assess the time lapse from Manuela's last meal and did the residue in her stomach match what she had eaten with her host family? Yes, and yes.

She was also able to state that Manuela had died about two hours after that meal. The gardaí now had a time line.

We dispersed and Manuela's body was returned to her mother and father.

The forensic science laboratory was busy processing all the exhibits from the scene. Unexpectedly a condom found at the scene provided vital evidence. Manuela's DNA profile was on the outside surface, so it had been used in her rape. Of course the DNA profile from the inner surface would identify the man who had raped and killed her. All that was needed now was a suspect.

The forensic laboratory was one step ahead: the unknown DNA profile from the condom was a match for a profile generated in a recent rape case. Gerald Barry was the suspect in the rape of a French woman eight weeks earlier. Criminals are sometimes not as clever as they like to think.

As in Pass the Parcel, we sent our individual findings around the circle, but instead of stripping something away, the parcel of evidence got larger and larger. The music stopped when it reached the DPP: would he or she look at what they had and drop it to the floor, game over, or nod, the music start again and the parcel move to judge and jury?

At court, we heard the one version we had not heard before: the defendant's. We could do no more. The jury had to decide. Gerald Barry was found guilty of the murder of Manuela Riedo.

Throughout the trial Manuela's mother and father were present. They had sent their daughter to Ireland to improve her English and now they were in court listening to the sordid details of the last few minutes of her life. It was humbling to meet them and express my sympathy for their loss, the loss of their 'angel'. They presented all of us with a small porcelain figurine of an angel lest we forget Manuela. Mine looks down on me as I sit at my desk, a constant reminder of the fragility of life.

Manuela's mother and father set up the Manuela Riedo Foundation in Ireland to raise awareness of and prevent sexual crime in the country. It helps to fund charities and agencies who provide support to victims of rape and sexual violence. Shame on us: they lost a Swiss angel and we gained vital services for victims of sexual assault.

8

Courts and Inquests

IN THE 1990S THERE WAS a cluster of prostitute deaths in the Glasgow area, resulting in talk of a serial killer rampaging through the city and fears that another 'Bible John' was on the loose. Bible John had roamed the Barrowland dance hall in Glasgow in the late 1960s, picking up women, who were later found dead, battered, strangled and sexually assaulted. He was so-called because the people who had been with the victims could describe the attacker, gave his name as John and said he was wont to quote from the Bible, decrying adulterous females attending such venues.

Despite a massive manhunt, the police never identified him. There were several suspects but no evidence to identify the murderer with any certainty. I became involved many years later, as the forensic pathologist acting for the Crown Office. In the mid-1990s, advances in DNA analysis meant that the police began reviewing unsolved cases where there was a possibility that stored evidence could identify a perpetrator. Of course, rape and rape-homicides offered the best chance of success as semen was often deposited on the victim during the course of the assault.

One of the suspects in the Bible John murders was John McInnes. He fitted the general description and was said to have been sighted in the Barrowland. He had been included in identification parades but had not been picked out by women who had come forward with information about the man last seen with the murder victims. The police believed that circumstantial evidence linked John McInnes to the murder of one of the victims, Helen Puttock. He had committed suicide in 1980, which might account for the sudden end to the reign of terror in the Barrowland.

In 1993 the death of Helen Puttock was reviewed. A semen stain had been identified on her clothing in 1968 at the time of the original investigation but now technology enabled a DNA profile to be obtained. John McInnes's siblings were informed of the ongoing investigation and consented to swabs being taken from them for analysis. The experts were of the opinion that there was sufficient similarity between the siblings' profiles and the semen stain to proceed with the investigation into John McInnes's role in the Barrowland deaths. A decision was made to exhume his body and take samples for DNA analysis.

Professor Tony Busuttil was observing proceedings on behalf of the family of the deceased and I was the forensic pathologist for the Crown. Exhumations are usually scheduled for dawn, or thereabouts, an unearthly hour, but the hope is that we can get in and out as quickly as possible, in particular before the press are alerted to our activity. On the appointed day we convened in the graveyard early to discuss our plan of action. A tent was erected over the grave site and the police commenced the excavation. These are very difficult operations. The adjacent gravesites must not be disturbed, which makes it difficult to access the grave of interest. There are also variables, which will compound the difficulty: how many bodies are in the grave, their order of interment, when the body was interred, the state of the coffin and the soil conditions.

In this instance we had to dig down a considerable distance to access the relevant coffin. The first contained the body of Mrs McInnes, John's mother, who had died seven years after her son. All care was taken that this coffin was recovered intact and removed to the funeral parlour, awaiting reinterment. The excavation continued until the next coffin was struck. Neither I nor Tony is particularly tall and I had to be lowered into the grave to confirm that we were dealing with the correct coffin and body. Tony elected to remain at the graveside but even this was hazardous and he found himself slipping into the hole, grabbed at the last second by police.

Manoeuvring a coffin out of a grave is difficult as the clearance is only a few centimetres but eventually we were successful. The remains were removed to the mortuary and bone samples were taken, the best source of material for DNA analyses given the time frame. Unfortunately, despite our best efforts, the laboratory could not get a full profile and the results were described as inconclusive. The Barrowland serial killer had not been identified and remains unidentified to this day.

Back to the deaths in the 1990s. Now the press was reporting the possibility of another serial killer in Glasgow. However, the only link between the victims was their employment. Of six women killed, four of the deaths got to court but only one trial ended in a conviction, twenty years after the death; two trials ended with a 'not proven' verdict and one with 'not guilty'. These were vicious and violent murders. I gave evidence in the trials, mindful, as always, that I was there as an expert to explain to the court how the victims had died and offer my opinion as to the circumstances of the death.

On one occasion I finished giving my evidence and, after cross-examination and re-examination by the barristers for the defence and the prosecution, I was excused. At this time the criminal courts were being renovated and the trials were held in a building that had been converted for the purpose. It had previously been a bank, luxuriously appointed in its time, all marble floors and pillars. As I made my way through the court, heading for the sturdy wooden doors leading out into the entrance hall, I was aware of my heels making a clicking sound as I walked across the marble floor.

Suddenly I became aware that this sound was

echoing and increasing in volume. I looked over my shoulder to see that the friends of the deceased were following me out *en masse*. I quickened my pace, fearing that some part of my evidence might have enraged the women and that retribution might follow. I got to the door but its hefty weight meant it took valuable seconds to push through it and out into the reception area. That was enough time for the women to catch up with me.

We poured out into the hall in a tight group. I looked around for any policemen who could come to my rescue. But, surprisingly, instead of angry rebukes my hand was grabbed and shaken while they thanked me for handling the findings so sensitively. As they left, one turned and said, 'I don't know how you do that job.' There was no answer to that. It was now official – I had a job that prostitutes thought was awful.

Despite the differing legal systems, the court services in Scotland and Ireland in criminal cases are very similar: a death has occurred, the findings support that someone is responsible for the death, a case is prepared for the prosecution, someone is charged with murder or manslaughter and their defence team disputes some or all of the evidence against the accused. There is probably a lot more to it than that, but that's it in a nutshell.

My role is as an expert witness to the court. I am unbiased and independent. I work with the police but not for the police. The coroner, similarly independent, has asked me to assist in the investigation of a death and the result of my postmortem examination will help determine the direction the investigation takes, whether the police prepare a case for the Director of Public Prosecutions (DPP) (Ireland), the Procurator Fiscal (Scotland) or the Criminal Prosecution Service (CPS) (England and Wales), or the case is referred back to the coroner and an inquest is held. If the former, the prosecution service will decide whether or not there is sufficient evidence to charge an individual, or individuals, with causing the death and if they should stand trial. If there is insufficient evidence to charge a particular individual or the evidence gathered shows there is no case to answer, the death will revert back to the coroner for a public inquiry. Either way the findings will be aired and the family will be appraised of the cause and circumstances of the death. In Scotland, there is no inquest and the case remains on hold for that day there is sufficient evidence.

The difference between a court hearing and a coroner's inquest is that the coroner cannot apportion blame to an individual, or an institution, even if the death is a murder. That can be particularly frustrating to the family of the deceased if the DPP decides there is insufficient evidence to proceed with a criminal trial and the family feel that justice has not been served.

The mantra of the criminal justice system is that it serves to protect the innocent and fairly convict the guilty; there is a fear of wrong or unfair conviction. A tall order. The onus is on the police, the courts and those giving evidence to ensure that what is presented in court is factual and robust, and can stand up to scrutiny. Remember the concept of innocent until proven guilty. The decision to charge a person with committing a crime, especially a murder, is not taken lightly. An incredible amount of work is put into collating evidence and interviewing witnesses. It takes months, if not years, to get a case into court. In Scotland a time limit is put on a trial date once someone is formally charged with murder.

Before I left Glasgow for Dublin at the beginning of 1998 the prosecution had 110 days to start the trial from the day the person accused of the crime was remanded in custody. This was to ensure justice without undue delay, and put considerable strain on the system: three months to gather the evidence and complete forensic investigations. In more recent years the preparation for trials has become more complex so in 2005 the 110-day rule was extended to 140 days, but even that is difficult to adhere to. The rule was necessary to prevent accused persons languishing in prison for lengthy periods before trial: most were remanded in custody once charged, unlike in Ireland where bail for serious crime is more common. Although the individual on bail may have to comply with strict rules, they are still at liberty and probably in no hurry to get into court. Innocent until proven guilty . . .

The system in the UK and Ireland is adversarial rather than inquisitorial, the European system. There are two sides to the story, maybe more. The prosecution presents their case and the defence, acting for the accused, will question the evidence presented.

The prosecution will set the scene, using photographs and maps of the area where the deceased was injured or killed. Then they will set out the circumstances leading up to the death:

who the victim was with, what they did, where they went, what happened. Eye-witnesses will be asked to give evidence to the court only of what they saw and heard, not what others told them: the Hearsay Rule. Giving evidence can be a daunting experience, even for the experts. The witness box is a lonely place. Many witnesses will never have been in a court before. Very often this is the first time in court for the person on trial in a murder case. They often look stunned to be there: that was not what they'd had in mind when they went out for a few drinks with their friends.

No matter whether you're called as a witness for the prosecution or for the defence, it is important to stick to the facts and not deviate from the statement you made: to do so will cause consternation in the court – the pleasant barrister guiding you through your evidence morphs into your worst nightmare. Unfortunately, due to the length of time it may take a case to get to court, memories will normally be a little fuzzy and, left to their own devices, the witness may have forgotten or misremembered the events of a particular night. Always best to say that you cannot remember, rather than fabricate the happenings, even if you're just trying to be helpful. There will be a statement you made to the police in the days following the incident and this can be used by counsel to prompt you or refresh your memory. Good honest citizens sometimes try too hard to be helpful, but this is neither the time nor the place for that. There may also be witnesses with a different agenda, who deliberately cause confusion and even lie. They will be dealt with by the courts. The truth will find you out.

A few witnesses relish the experience of standing on a raised dais, the centre of attention, the court hanging on every word. In one case I was asked to be in court at a particular time to give evidence. When I arrived I was told a witness was just finishing off, did I mind waiting? I settled into a seat at the back of the court, not too interested in what the civilian witness was saying. He was part through describing to the prosecution barrister what he had seen on the night of the incident. I was very impressed: he was self-assured, clear and precise about what he had seen and heard. I found myself quite engaged by the young man. A very credible witness, I thought.

The defence barrister got to his feet and proceeded with the cross-examination of the witness, who, by the account he had just given, was eye-witness to the fatal incident. The defence barrister tried to find some little discrepancy or chink of doubt in the man's story. The witness remained steadfast in his account of what he had seen and heard. All was going fairly well until he felt the need to embellish his account, not regarding the actions leading to the death but to the 'discussion' he had allegedly had with the accused party, adding a few expletives into the alleged conversation. Coming from Glasgow where expletives are rather common in daily talk, this didn't ring alarm bells with me. But in the context of one person threatening another, it can increase the perceived level of threat. 'This fucking rain is awful' is not quite as frightening as 'I'm gonna fuckin' kill ya.' Rightly, the defence pounced on the change of emphasis in the alleged exchange between the two parties. The witness was asked to explain why this part of the dialogue had not been referred to in his original statement or mentioned in court earlier. 'I don't know,' was his rather weak response. His credibility had been questioned and his standing as a reliable witness was dented. Stick to the facts.

Now that we have got to the part in the trial where we have an account, or at least a version, of the events leading up to the death, it is time to introduce the witnesses who will give evidence as to the cause of death (the forensic pathologist) and the evidence that links the accused with the deceased and the scene (the forensic scientists). The pathologist describes their findings at the postmortem, each and every injury, no matter how small, and which of the injuries caused the death. As an expert, the forensic pathologist is allowed to give their opinion on how the injuries were caused – for example, a punch, a kick, a fall or a blow from an object. They will often be cross-examined by the defence barrister. Sometimes this is just to clarify some points but it may be that the accused has given a slightly different version of the incident and the defence barrister wants to know if this is feasible.

On a few occasions the defence team will have their own forensic pathologist, who may have a different opinion on the circumstances, and sometimes even the cause, of the death. This is more common when death is due to head injuries. In such deaths the injuries sustained may be complex, as is the interpretation of how the injuries were sustained.

My duty is to the court and therefore I must ensure that my evidence is unbiased. This may mean that my evidence is more favourable to one side than the other, but I cannot make the facts fit the case. When a finding does not support the prosecution evidence, I must make that clear to the jury. It is for the jury to decide the outcome of a case based on all the evidence.

It is also not my role to sensationalise my findings: the facts should speak for themselves. While the prosecution may describe the events leading to a death as a frenzied attack, I try not to use inflammatory language. I am always mindful that the family of the deceased are in the court. You cannot shield them from the fact that a loved one has died but it serves no purpose to be over-dramatic or graphic. On one occasion a young man had been violently assaulted and died from head injuries. Five persons were standing trial for their parts in the death. I was of the opinion that the severe injuries were due to blows from a blunt object. The man's scalp was split in several places, his skull badly fractured, his brain bruised and torn. I described the injuries in a matter-of-fact way, horrific as they were. The judge was appalled. 'The skull was broken up into tiny pieces?'

'Yes, Your Honour, a comminuted fracture of the skull, like a jigsaw puzzle.'

'And these were *driven* into the brain?'

'Well, as a result of the blows the brain was badly injured,' I countered.

At this point one of the defence barristers asked the judge for an adjournment as his client was feeling a little unwell. I suspect most of the court was a little queasy. When we returned, the defence council informed the judge that his client was pleading guilty. I guess the judge's apparent shock at the injuries sustained by the deceased was also felt by one of the accused. The others held out and the trial continued. I can but hope that at least that young man had learned his lesson and was successfully rehabilitated in prison.

I am not a lawyer, and have never aspired to become one, but people seem to assume that I must have a certain knowledge of the law. Sorry to disappoint, but there is danger in having one foot in the forensic-pathology camp and the other in the legal camp. We are completely different animals with completely different roles.

The forensic pathologist owes allegiance to the court, independent and unbiased, while the lawyers have picked a side, prosecuting or defending, and their allegiance is to their client: the state or the person accused of the crime. As part of my role to explain to the court what happened to the deceased person and the cause of their death, it behoves me to discuss this with the opposing parties.

In Scotland, the prosecuting and defending barristers would have a discussion with the forensic pathologist at some time prior to the trial, on separate occasions, to gain an understanding of what exactly the pathologist thinks happened, and whether or not that is either helpful or detrimental to the prosecution or defence position. It makes no odds to me either way: my role is neither to prosecute nor defend an individual accused of murder but to 'tell the truth, the whole truth and nothing but the truth' of how this deceased died and why I think it is a murder.

In Ireland discussions with counsel are less formal, often a quick chat during a trial, just before I go into the witness box. This makes it vital that my original postmortem report is detailed and comprehensive: anyone should be able to pick it up and understand the salient details. That is why it is essential that all cases, and the subsequent reports produced, are peer-reviewed by at least one colleague. This not only ensures that simple mistakes, such as mixing up left from right when describing injuries, are not missed, that spelling and grammar are correct, but, most importantly, that the reasoning behind the conclusions is challenged and tested so that the final report is factual, accurate and will stand up to questioning in court.

When I first went to court in Ireland, after thirteen years of defending my position in court in Scotland, I was amazed that my evidence went unchallenged, the court accepting my version of events without question. A curt thank-you and I was dismissed. I should have been relieved but I was perturbed: I am only human, and humans make mistakes.

The 'humans' in the court were, to my mind, making a monumental mistake in assuming an expert witness is infallible. What if I was wrong? There is only one person who professes to be infallible and only on certain matters, and not everyone accepts that. But the central criminal court in Ireland was putting its trust in some wee blonde woman from Glasgow that they didn't know from Adam – or Eve, for that matter. You have to earn respect and I was very conscious that I was an unknown quantity. Just because I was the deputy state pathologist did not mean I was an expert in forensic pathology. I had been tried

Marie Cassidy

and tested in Scotland and had earned the title of expert, but not in Ireland.

I decided to speak to the DPP about my concerns regarding this blanket acceptance of everything I said. The then state pathologist Jack Harbison thought I had taken leave of my senses: he could not understand why I would offer myself up to be questioned by anyone, prosecution or defence. But that was precisely what I wanted: if there was any chance that I was mistaken in some of my assertions about how someone had died, the court had to be made aware that there might be another version of events.

Although I spent days, weeks and months, on occasion, mulling over and checking facts, and eventually reached certain conclusions, could I 'swear' in court that this was the whole truth? Perhaps there was information I was not aware of, or a version of events that the defence had not had the opportunity to test if they had not been afforded the chance to test my opinion. The DPP accepted the flaw in the system but took pains to point out that if the prosecuting counsel had a little chat with me to clarify my findings prior to my giving evidence then the defence would expect the same.

- 338 -

Exactly! They always say 'be careful what you wish for', but this wasn't about me showing the court how clever I was, this was about justice, or fairness. Potentially someone's liberty could be at stake. It is essential that we get it right. Nowadays, with the introduction of mandatory peer review, all cases will have been discussed at a case-review meeting, and the postmortem reports will have been read by one or two colleagues before the final report is sent to the coroner. This ensures that the pathology evidence is tested before the case goes to court so when the pathologist appears in court he or she is confident that their evidence can withstand a rigorous cross-examination by the defence counsel.

England and Wales have a long tradition of pre-trial conferences, which streamlines criminal trials. The forensic pathologists acting for the prosecution and defence discuss the relevant facts and findings before a murder trial and agree common ground. When the case comes to trial both sides know what is agreed and what issues the pathologists disagree over. Usually these are the most contentious trials, often involving head injuries causing the deaths of adults and children. In Scotland the legal system differs from England, Wales and Ireland, as two pathologists will examine the body of a murder victim. This should ensure less chance of error in the pathology evidence.

In the majority of murder trials, the pathology evidence is not contentious and is not challenged. The cause of death is not in dispute. For the defence team it may be a case of damage limitation, particularly if there are multiple injuries. Their contention is that of the many, only one was fatal, the others irrelevant to the death of that poor individual. I don't think juries are fooled by such courtroom antics.

It is rare that the pathologist states in court something unexpected, but it can happen. If the pathologist was not made aware of certain evidence, or the defence version of events, they may, on some occasions, have to revise their opinion. This can cause consternation in the middle of a trial, which is why it's better to chat before we go into court. No one wants a case ambushed. It is not in anyone's interest, prosecution or defence.

I still find it incredible that some barristers don't understand the role of the expert, the prosecution adopting me as their witness against the accused, and the defence assuming I am the enemy. Even more galling are the experts who don't understand their role: no matter who pays them, their duty is to the court. In the majority of homicides, if someone is charged with the death they have the right to demand that a second postmortem examination is carried out as part of their defence strategy, to determine the facts of the death. This ensures that the defence knows what they are defending. They are informed by the police of what their client is charged with, but not the finer details: the number of injuries; injuries that support a defence of self-defence; a pattern of trauma that supports their client's version of events.

The full postmortem report will take weeks to complete and the defence must prepare their case, so having as much information as early as possible is in the interest of their client. The second pathologist is also a safeguard against the first pathologist giving a biased opinion, favouring the prosecution, without considering alternative explanations. This should not happen so often now but occasionally it does. The pathologist giving the second opinion is usually from outside the jurisdiction or an independent practitioner within it.

The difficulty with the right to have a second examination is that it delays the body's return to the family. In Ireland there is an unwritten rule of five working days, introduced relatively recently by Dr Brian Farrell when he was the Dublin City Coroner. In Scotland the body would usually be retained for a week or two; arrests were either prompt or it was accepted that the investigation could take months and therefore the body should be returned. In England and Wales bodies were sometimes retained for months, awaiting completion of an investigation, a real hardship for families, but this has been remedied in part by the coroner instructing a second postmortem examination to be carried out in the event of a protracted investigation so that the families can make arrangements for a funeral.

I would give opinions on murder cases in Northern Ireland. If the pathologist carrying out the first postmortem is an experienced forensic pathologist, it is rare that the second would find that something had been overlooked, but sometimes the findings are open to interpretation. If there is a difference of opinion between the pathologists it is best that it is known to the court. This gives both pathologists an opportunity to revise their findings and, if necessary, their opinion.

This is in the interest of the court. I have been

ambushed by the defence when they have had a report prepared by another pathologist and there is some difference of opinion, which I have not been made aware of until I'm being cross-examined. The problem is that a sentence taken out of context can have a different meaning and is not necessarily a true reflection of the other pathologist's opinion. In those cases I have to explain to the court that I was not aware of this report so need time to read and consider its findings.

Usually in those circumstances the difference between us has been trivial and, when considered in the context of the evidence before the court, makes no substantive difference to my evidence and opinion. Sometimes the defence just wants to muddy the waters. I am always open to considering an alternative opinion – I have to be prepared to change mine if necessary. Remember, I have sworn to tell the truth, the whole truth and nothing but the truth.

More annoying is the pathologist whose opinion is that my evidence is wrong. They offer no alternative explanation, just assert that I am wrong in my interpretation. At the end of the day, my opinion is based on my interpretation of my findings at postmortem, in the context of the circumstances and other evidence. I fully accept there may be an alternative scenario, and would be willing to consider it, if such was offered. Even worse is the pathologist who confuses, or misleads, the court by appearing to offer an alternative explanation but in reality does not.

In Glasgow a young woman was gunned down at her home. She was found dead lying on the stairs leading up to the flats above hers. She had been shot in the mouth and a bullet lodged in her tongue. This had not killed her, and there was a trail of blood from her flat and up two flights of stairs, presumably from when she attempted to get help from her neighbours, then back down to the landing below where she was found collapsed. Her boyfriend alleged he had returned home to find her collapsed but still alive. She was dead by the time the emergency services arrived. The police immediately declared it a crime scene and the relevant parties were asked to attend, including myself and the forensic team.

Sally Cannon was covered with blood and a preliminary examination showed an injury behind her ear; a detailed examination in the mortuary confirmed a further two gunshot wounds to her head, a total of three altogether. We walked through the scene in her footsteps, following the trail of her blood, imagining her panic, seriously injured and frightened for her life, desperately seeking help.

The postmortem was intriguing. There were three gunshot wounds to her head: one bullet was recovered from her tongue and one from inside her skull; the third was lying free in the hole in her skull. Bullets may be tiny but as they strike their target at high velocity a massive amount of energy is dissipated through the body. The small holes I find on the surface of the body often belie the devastating internal injuries. It is these injuries that cause death, either due to destruction of the vital organs or vast quantities of blood lost.

This woman had lost a considerable quantity of blood, but not sufficient to be solely responsible for her death. Despite the injury to her tongue, the major source of blood loss, she had not choked on blood; there was a gaping hole in her skull where two bullets had struck but, apart from a little bruising on the surface of the brain, there was no haemorrhage into the brain or extensive bleeding inside the skull cavity, nothing obvious to cause rapid death.

The bullets appeared to have come to a grinding

halt as soon as they hit tissue. The gun used was obviously a low-velocity weapon, a handgun, which was never recovered. She was a drug user but otherwise she was relatively healthy. While her death was obviously due to gunshot trauma to the head, what was the mechanism? A pathological conundrum.

The forensic scientists examined the scene, her clothing and her boyfriend's. They came to the conclusion that all the blood at the scene was from her; that she had been ambulant after being injured, most likely after she was shot in the mouth; and that she was likely shot in the head where her body was found. This was consistent with my interpretation. The examination of her clothing did not advance that theory. The examination of the boyfriend's clothes revealed a blood-spatter pattern made up of tiny droplets of blood, which the scientists thought was due to the back-spatter caused when a bullet strikes tissue, the force tearing the tissues apart as it burrows into them, causing blood to spray back towards anything, or anyone, close to the injured party.

Their interpretation of this was that the boyfriend had been close to her when she was shot and therefore, as he had stated no one was there when he found her, he had shot her. The defence argued that the blood-spatter pattern was caused as he cradled her after he found her because she had coughed blood over him before she died.

The case came to court. We all gave evidence. I tried to explain how the gunshot injuries had caused her death and proposed that the shock wave through the brain, caused by the bullet striking the skull and its kinetic injury dissipating through the brain tissue, could have a similar effect to a lightning strike if the brainstem, the central powerhouse, was in its path, essentially causing it to short-circuit. The net effect of this could be instant cardio-respiratory arrest.

This explanation was troublesome to the defence: if she had died almost instantly after she was shot on the side of her head she would not have been coughing when her boyfriend found her, which negated their explanation for the blood-spatter on his clothing. I knew that, by proposing this mechanism for her death, I would be attacked vehemently by the defence. These are the moments in the witness box you fear, when you know that your evidence is going to scupper the defence case.

I used to pray for divine intervention or at least for the judge to tell the defence to stop badgering the witness. But usually I just had to plough on and try to keep composed. It was at times like these that I wondered why I did this for a living. The mantra is to tell the truth, explain your reasoning, and at the end of the day leave it to the jury to decide whether or not they agree with the evidence in totality.

The defence questioning was challenging but I survived. What the jury and the public don't know is that the forensic pathologists and the barristers are actually friends who respect one another. I never took the questioning of my evidence personally: we all have a role to play in the justice system and we must all act in the best interest of justice. But justice for one is not necessarily justice for another. I prefer fairness, and I have always tried to be a fair witness. That has been recognised by barristers on both sides, but it would not be fair if they did not test my evidence. That goes with the territory. The case continued, we all said our piece, the prosecution and defence made their closing arguments and the judge summarised the evidence.

In many of the murder trials I have been involved in, the defendant is not required to give evidence. Whether they do or not is a decision made by the defence team. This will, of course, depend on the defence position. If the argument is that the person accused of the crime says they were not there and did not do it, they would have nothing relevant to say.

One of the most experienced defence barristers in Scotland, Donald Findlay, had an interesting tactic in such cases: as soon as I walked into the witness box, he would stand, making sure everyone noticed, and exit the court, gown flapping behind him. He was making the point that he had no interest in the upsetting details in my report as the matter had nothing to do with his client. I usually heaved a sigh of relief because I knew there would be no awkward questioning of my evidence.

The beauty of working for the defence is that you get access to all of the evidence, not just what the prosecution thinks is relative to the case, but also the 'schedule of unused material'. I get boxes and boxes of statements, which I would never see when called by the prosecution. This also includes the statements that the prosecution has decided they are not going to use. It can take me days, but I am presented with the whole picture, and I get to decide what is relevant to the death, not to the prosecution or defence cases. These can make harrowing reading, particularly in domestic-abuse cases where there may have been months of abuse, physical, emotional and sexual, leading up to the death of one of the parties.

It can be hard as an expert to remain unbiased when, as an ordinary citizen, having read the disturbing facts of the events leading up to the death, your instinct is that 'He should be locked away for ever' or 'Why didn't she kill him sooner?' But I'm not an ordinary citizen: even though I can appreciate the arguments for either party, my role is to make sure the evidence is fair, particularly the pathology evidence.

One thing I find amazing is reading the police interviews with the defendant. Through a number of interviews they are steadfast in answering, 'No comment,' to every question asked. They are questioned on the hours or days leading up to the murder, who they were with, what everyone is saying. The details of the murder are put to them; in some instances, photographs will be shown of the scene. 'No comment.' And then, a complete about-turn and they begin singing like the proverbial linty, chapter and verse. What makes them cave in? Do they have a conscience? Or has their lawyer told them, 'The game's a bogey', the facts speak for themselves, the evidence is stacked against you? I always think, You could probably have held out for one more interview. But the truth will out.

Meanwhile in Glasgow the jury returned a 'guilty of murder' verdict, and off went the boyfriend to prison for 'life'. The end. No, this is not the end. There are some who accept their sentence and go quietly, but many do not, particularly if facing life in prison for murder. Some will claim that they did not get a fair trial, others maintain their innocence. The prosecution and the police feel they have done a good job, and are probably delighted with the sentence handed down, as are the family of the victim. All believe justice has been done. It might have been. But it might not. The defence team may cite an error of law and that the judge was unfair in his or her summing up, particularly if they have not explained to the jury the defence of self-defence or the partial defences of loss of control, provocation or diminished responsibility, which would have allowed them to consider a charge of manslaughter (culpable homicide in Scotland) rather than murder.

The person convicted may be very unhappy with his defence team, arguing that they failed to defend him robustly enough. That there has been a miscarriage of justice due to certain evidence being improperly allowed by the judge, or evidence disallowed, which might have affected the outcome. Or that the weight of the evidence does not support the verdict.

As regards the death of the young woman in Glasgow, the boyfriend convicted of her murder appealed against his conviction on the basis that he had been inadequately defended, citing that his defence team had not called their own experts to rebut the forensic evidence given in court. Appeals against criminal convictions are rarely successful, but a review of the case concluded that he had not had a fair trial: his conviction was quashed and a date was set for a retrial.

Six years after the first trial we were back in court. By then I was deputy state pathologist in Ireland, and when I was given notice of the trial I was in Sierra Leone recovering bodies for the UN. I was flown home via Paris to Edinburgh. Unfortunately, the nature of the work in Sierra Leone meant that I had only the clothes I was travelling in, the rest left behind. In the airport in Paris I had to buy clothes suitable for court; the choice was limited but anything was better than what I had on. After travelling for twenty-four hours I was met at the airport by the police and taken straight to court to give evidence. Not ideal circumstances.

On that occasion the new defence team had no intention of disappointing their client and was going to ensure that their performance was more than adequate. The tone of the cross-examination was fiercely adversarial. My evidence was vigorously rebuffed by defence counsel and they had a pathologist who was categorically of the opinion that I was wrong in my interpretation of the mechanism of death. Death due to a head injury was not instantaneous, as I had asserted: it took some time for the brain to cease functioning and the person to die so it was highly likely that she was still alive when discovered by her boyfriend.

I agreed, as I had in the first trial, that this was an unusual case. While I also agreed that normally death in a head injury was due to the extent of injury to the brain or compression of it by haemorrhaging inside the skull, I reiterated that there was no evidence of either. The forensic scientist who gave evidence at the first trial got a similar grilling. The defence position was to undermine the evidence presented by the witnesses called by the prosecution. There was no doubt to anyone in the court that this time around the defence team had defended with vigour and the witnesses, including myself, left the box battered and bruised.

At the end of the trial the new jury retired to consider the evidence presented. On this occasion they returned with a verdict of 'not proven', a uniquely Scottish verdict: the evidence was not sufficient to convict but there was some doubt about the innocence of the defendant. After spending some years in prison, the defendant was allowed to leave the court a free man, but not an innocent one.

It is my role as an expert witness to present my evidence to the court, in particular the jury, in such a manner that they not only get the facts but can follow how I reached certain opinions. Having spent six years at medical school mastering the Latin terminology, on day one in forensic pathology I was told to ditch it and revert to understandable English. My reports are long and detailed – there may be dozens and dozens of injuries, external and internal. I am mindful that the descriptions are long-winded and that the jury will find it tedious having to concentrate on the minutiae of every bruise, graze, stab wound, gunshot injury or laceration.

During the course of my postmortem examination every mark is photographed. Every picture tells a story, and every postmortem photograph tells its unique story. It would be so much easier to show the jury select photographs to illustrate my descriptions, but the counsel for the defence argue that these would be prejudicial to the defendant. Hello! The defendant is standing trial for murder: am I missing something?

In order to illustrate how difficult it is to concentrate when listening to a forensic pathologist giving lengthy testimony without any illustration – a photograph, diagram or drawing – I tested this with a class of medical students. Surely they would at least have a grasp of simple medical terminology and anatomy. Each student was given a sheet of paper with the outline of a human head and neck, and I then read out part of a postmortem report. I had recently given evidence in this case at the Old Bailey in London.

The murder had happened in Ireland and the perpetrator had fled the country. To cut a long story short, he was eventually apprehended and elected to stand trial in the UK as he was a British citizen. It had been a brutal murder of a young woman, who was stabbed multiple times. What made the case interesting was the placement of the stab wounds to her neck. Rather than random, haphazardly arranged wounds, such as you would expect in a struggle, the stab wounds to the back of her neck were very precise in their location. The blade of a knife had penetrated the skin and soft tissues over the cervical spine and between the individual vertebrae into the spinal canal to partly sever the spinal cord. This suggested that her assailant had had some medical knowledge.

That was an important point as the person standing trial for the murder had a medical background so it was essential that the jury understood the significance of where those injuries were and their effects. Diagrams were used in court to good effect, and the prosecution was successful in gaining a conviction.

In our mini research project, the medical students were asked to listen to a description of twelve of the stab wounds to the head and neck in this case and to plot them on the diagram they had been given. So far so good.

Oh dear! The results were disappointing. The majority managed to plot twelve stab wounds on the diagram but the anatomical locations varied widely, and only about a tenth of the class correctly identified the location of all the stab wounds.

The second part of the experiment was to determine whether or not an illustration of wounds would improve the understanding of the oral evidence. The students were shown colour photographs, black-and-white photographs, diagrams and an artist's impression of the injuries, then asked to rank them in the order in which they thought a jury might find most helpful.

The majority found the photographs disturbing and preferred the diagrams. Such sensitive souls, our trainee doctors. I hope they toughened up before they were let loose in the big bad world. The point is, if medical students had difficulty without illustrations, juries must find it impossible at times. I tend to watch the jury closely when I'm giving evidence. I look for what I call 'nodding dog syndrome', checking that they are engaged and following the points. Sometimes I notice a puzzled expression and have to try to explain something in a slightly different way, looking for the nod that tells me they've got it. Occasionally, because I am watching the jury so intently, I have noticed jurors finding my evidence disturbing, evident in their extreme pallor and slumped position, and have brought it to the attention of the court. Thankfully, most made a full recovery; one was whisked off in an ambulance, but the judge decided we could continue one man down.

Once all the witnesses have given evidence in a criminal trial the jury have to decide, taking into consideration the entire body of evidence, whether the defendant is innocent or guilty. It is an onerous task.

In many cases the evidence against a person is so overwhelming and damning that a guilty verdict is inevitable, but sometimes there may be an element of doubt. It is in these latter cases that the verdict cannot be predicted with certainty: it depends on the deliberations of the jury, supposedly a cross-section of society. Unlike the trials in the USA, where jury selection is an art, in the UK and Ireland it is more pot-luck. Jurors are randomly selected from the electoral register.

Many will try to avoid jury service so certain sectors of society will not be represented. On the day, the potential jurors amass at court and, again, are randomly selected for whatever cases are commencing. Fear not, a private investigator has not been rummaging around in your murky past: your skeletons are safe in your closet. Generally, if the barristers like the look of you, you're in, if not, you're out, but they must give a valid reason for challenging your selection. Jury selection takes hours, not days.

The rewards for your trouble are meagre, basic travel allowance, about five pounds for your lunch and a paltry sum for loss of earnings, about sixty pounds per day in the UK. In Ireland you get your lunch. Not much recompense for deciding the fate of someone accused of committing murder. And they wonder why people desperately try to get out of their civic duty! But it is still difficult to come to the decision that the person sitting in the dock was capable of committing the crime that has been described, in awful detail, over the last few days or weeks.

The criminal courts, in particular, are over-subscribed: a court or even a judge may be unavailable, and a case may have to be deferred until there is a vacant slot. Sometimes important witnesses do not turn up or a guilty plea is entered at the last minute. At least as a juror you may be off the hook, but think of the accused and the witnesses who turned up for the trial only to be told they will have to come back another day.

Sometimes it will be a 'done deal': the evidence is overwhelmingly convincing that the defendant is guilty. At other times there may be some dissent in the jury room. If the jury cannot reach a unanimous agreement the judge may accept a majority verdict. Otherwise it may be back to the drawing board. The pressure on this disparate group of people, with their different backgrounds and life experiences, to come to a unanimous decision is enormous: guilty or not guilty, black or white.

But life is not so easily defined, and neither is murder, which is why I always thought that the Scottish third alternative was a good decision: 'not proven', meaning insufficient evidence to convict or exonerate so there is an element of doubt. It may be seen as a cop-out but I was usually not surprised when this verdict was returned in some murder trials as I agreed that the evidence was not 100 per cent conclusive. The main problem with that verdict was that the defendant could not be retried. I can understand why the relatives of a murder victim would be highly disappointed and angered by it: to them, it was more or less an innocent verdict. The person who had been accused of this heinous crime did not get a prison sentence; justice was not done.

On a cold and wet Friday night in 1992 I was

contacted by the police regarding a suspicious death in Hamilton, about fifteen miles from Glasgow. The body of a young woman had been found in undergrowth in a car park near Marks & Spencer in the town centre. Off I set to the scene. It was dark and access to the body was difficult. She was well tucked into the bushes and it looked as if she must have been dragged in: she hadn't just fallen back into the shrubbery, nor would she have been likely to venture in voluntarily. She was lying on her back and her clothing was in disarray, her lower garments missing.

It was difficult to make out individual injuries in the poor lighting but her face appeared dark and was covered with blood, and twigs seemed to be sticking out of her nose. Mindful of losing forensic evidence by trampling over the scene, it was decided that the best course of action was to get the body out of there and into the mortuary as quickly as possible. This had all the hallmarks of a sex-related homicide. If so, time was of the essence. I wanted to get the examination under way to gather the forensic evidence that might help identify her attacker. In Scotland, as two pathologists were required to perform the postmortem, I rang Dr Walter Spilg, my on-call colleague, apologising for the lateness of the hour, and asked him to join me in the city mortuary in Glasgow. We would work through the night.

Once we got the body into the bright light of the mortuary, the enormity of our task became obvious. She was injured beyond recognition. But, as with every case, we started at the top of her head and, over several hours, made our way down to her feet. Our task was to identify her, determine the cause of death and gather the forensic evidence.

We struck lucky with the identity as she had a student card, with the name Amanda Duffy and a photograph. Unfortunately, due to the injuries sustained, we could not be certain that this was her because the skin on her face was badly grazed and was now dark brown, and the shape of her face distorted and swollen. But the hair in the photograph was distinctive, long with tight curls, matching that of the body on the mortuary table. We were convinced that this was Amanda.

Her injuries were horrendous. She had been beaten about the head and there was damage to her neck, indicating that it had been compressed, by a hand, arm or even a foot. Her death could have been due to the head or neck injuries, but probably to the combined effects of both. This was indeed a brutal assault. Her state of undress and the pattern of injuries were consistent with this having been a sexually motivated murder. A complicating factor was that the body had been mutilated after death and twigs had been forced into the nose, mouth and vagina. I had never seen anything like it before, and even Walter, who was an old hand, was very quiet. I was hands-on and he was taking the notes.

The mood in the mortuary was sombre. Weekends there were normally spent dealing with gangland killings and domestics. This was not normal. This was a young woman who, only hours earlier, had been celebrating the next step in her life, and someone had taken that life from her in a most brutal way. We were gathered around her, as if trying to keep her safe. It was too late for that. We did what we do best: we made sure that everything was recorded and every stray hair or fibre was collected. If there was trace evidence that would help identify her killer, we would find it.

By morning we had done everything we could. There was only one thing left to do. During the examination we had described an injury on one of her breasts, an unusual injury in an unusual site. I thought this might be a bite mark, which meant contacting the forensic dentist and getting him down to the mortuary. The next step would normally be to inform the family and ask a close relative to come to the mortuary to confirm that this was the body of Amanda Duffy, as we suspected.

In the majority of cases there would be no hesitation. No one wants that knock on the door first thing in the morning, or anytime, no one wants to have to go to a mortuary to identify a family member, but we must confirm the identity. We needed to be sure this was Amanda Duffy. The young woman's face was so badly injured that we were concerned she might not be who we thought she was. Students do tend to borrow identity cards, but if this was Amanda Duffy, what effect would it have on her parents to see her?

We decided to try to identify her by other means. The forensic dentist could also assist us by charting her teeth to compare with her dental records. He confirmed that this was the body of Amanda Duffy. He also confirmed that the injury on the breast was an aggressive bite – the skin was torn – and showed us the marks made by individual teeth on the skin. Such was the detail, he was able to provide a dental profile and made a cast of the bite, which would later positively identify the man charged with her murder. We had a cause of death; we had collected the trace evidence; we had identified the body positively by scientific means. What more could we have done?

On reflection, we could have been more empathetic towards Amanda's parents. Collectively we took the decision that it was best for the family to remember Amanda as she was, dressed for a night out, excited about her future prospects, rather than to carry the image of the battered and lifeless body lying on the mortuary table. A paternalistic attitude that we now recognise as not always in the best interest of the families concerned.

Over the years I have learned that it is not enough to be informed that a close family member has died: many wish to see for themselves; to touch, hold, kiss and cry over the body. We denied Amanda's family that right. Nowadays I will do everything I can to ensure that families have the chance to say their goodbyes in person. It is not always possible but even if all they can see and touch is a hand that is often enough.

Nowadays the APTs are trained in reconstruction and will do all in their power, as will the undertakers, but sometimes I have to bring in professional assistance. One APT in particular, Glyn Tallon, is incredibly skilled and I have called upon his services when there is severe head trauma or disfigurement due to postmortem changes that cause discoloration and swelling of the features. He is a master at employing techniques to conceal and disguise these and allow the families to view the body without being shocked by the changes in their loved one. This comes at a cost not everyone can bear, but Glyn is very generous with his time and has helped on several occasions, most recently when a husband killed his wife and concealed the body for several days. A combination of trauma and postmortem changes meant she was barely recognisable, but Glyn worked his magic and her family were able to view her.

Then Amanda's parents were dealt another blow. It would set them on a path that eventually led to a change in the law. When the case came to court, the man accused of her murder, Francis Auld, was known to her and she had been seen in his company that fateful night. He accepted that he had been with her but said that they had met up with another male and she had gone off with him. There was no disputing the cause of death. I outlined the injuries and how I thought she had come about them, then detailed the mutilation of the body. Even the defence counsel agreed that the death was horrific, but of course his client was not responsible. Surely only someone with a severe psychiatric history could have done such a thing and this man was sane. This is another defence ploy: normal, sane people do not do horrific things and therefore the person who committed the crime must have been deranged.

A damning piece of evidence was the bite on her breast. There was no doubt that the bite had been inflicted by the accused, which he did not deny, but I was amazed by the proposition that a young woman would have adjusted her clothing afterwards, then gone off with another male. There was no blood inside her bra to support this possibility. The forensic scientist confirmed this but also stated that hairs found at the scene matched the accused. The defence counsel, Donald Findlay, dismissed this as secondary transfer: the hairs had been transferred onto Amanda when they were in close contact and it was these hairs that were found at the scene and therefore the accused need not have been at the scene to shed them. The scientist accepted this. Once all the evidence had been presented the jury retired to deliberate. A verdict of 'not proven' was returned. The accused walked out of court.

Most people were amazed at the verdict but I'd had my doubts about getting a conviction. Donald Findlay had raised some doubts over the forensic science evidence, which was obviously enough to sway the jury. Amanda's parents must have been devastated: it had seemed, on the face of it, a straightforward case, with a foregone conclusion. The accused was still free and their daughter was dead.

That was not the end of the story. The Duffys continued to try for some redress. One course of action is to take a private prosecution against a person. This is not common but has happened in a few murder cases, such as the O.J. Simpson case in the States and the Stephen Lawrence murder in the UK. In 1995 the Duffys took a civil case against Francis Auld. The level of proof in a civil case is less than expected in a criminal court, probability versus beyond reasonable doubt, and Francis Auld was found to be responsible for Amanda Duffy's death and her parents were awarded £50,000. Of course, a civil court can only award damages. The Duffys never received any money.

Since the criminal trial Amanda's parents

campaigned tirelessly for a change in the law: the scrapping of the not-proven verdict. In 2011 the Double Jeopardy (Scotland) Act was passed, nearly twenty years after Amanda's death. Now a person can be tried twice for the same crime, but the 'not proven' verdict remains. Amanda's death was considered with a view to a second trial, but the evidence was ruled inadmissible. Francis Auld remained a free man. He died of cancer a few years later. Amanda's parents never had the closure, or justice, they and Amanda deserved.

As an expert witness I am painfully aware of the impact of my evidence. There is always the fear of an unfair or wrong conviction, but should that be at the expense of justice, or fairness, for the family of the deceased?

9

The 'Ologists

THE WOMAN HADN'T SEEN HER friend for a few days. They worked the same drag and a no-show meant no money. None of them could afford that, not just from the money point of view but the repercussions from their 'minder'. She gave it another night, and when her friend still hadn't appeared she decided to check her out. You never knew what could happen in their game. The flat was dark and quiet. Knocking and shouting had no effect. Sometimes you have to trust your gut instinct. She couldn't get in so decided she had to call the police, not a decision any of them would make lightly. The door was flimsy and it didn't take much of an effort for the police to gain entry.

To the untrained eye the state of the flat – bedsit, really – would have been enough to raise the alarm, but the police had seen it all before. Squalor is an unfortunate side-effect of drugs and prostitution. In the midst of the chaos they found the crumpled body of a young woman, semi-naked. She had been dead for at least a couple of days. The temperatures inside and outside the flat could only be described as cold. Money for a meter was never an option in these circumstances. The police were mentally filing this under 'drug-related death', but protocols had to be observed so an investigation was launched.

I saw what the police had seen, but with a slightly different eye. Many of the bruises on the young woman's limbs were probably a consequence of her lifestyle but not the mark around her neck. She had been strangled. The body was taken to the city mortuary and the cause of death was confirmed as ligature strangulation. She had been murdered.

We knew who she was, courtesy of her friend, we knew how she had died and that she had died in the flat. What we didn't know was who had killed her, even if we thought we knew why: sex or drugs. I wasn't going to solve that part of the puzzle. Reinforcements were needed, the forensic army, in all its various disguises: the 'ologists.

Who will answer, or assist in answering, the vital questions? Every murder investigation has different requirements. In the above case we took samples to try to establish the identity of the killer. But first we needed a list of potential suspects. A difficult task in this death. To narrow it down we had to establish when she had died, that old chestnut the 'time of death'. The best I could offer was that she had been dead for at least two days. After the first forty-eight hours the parameters we use to assist in calculating the interval since death are unreliable. Once circulation stops, the tissues become depleted of oxygen, which sets off a chain of chemical reactions that affect the muscle cells, causing them to stiffen. The bigger the muscle bundle, the longer this takes. Small muscles in the face and hands are first to become rigid. The wave of muscle stiffening slowly spreads through the entire body until, literally, the body is as stiff as a board.

Occasionally this can happen immediately, a state of instant rigor known as cadaveric spasm. Writers adore this possibility, 'found with the gun still grasped in his hand' or 'the dying man clutching at straws'. The most extreme example I have seen was a young man who died accidentally after inhaling hydrocarbon gas from a bell jar in a laboratory. He was as if frozen in time, standing upright but his upper half bent, his face hovering over the large glass jar on the bench top, his car keys still clutched in his right hand. When we moved the jar he remained in position: sudden cadaveric spasm associated with the sudden cardiac arrest from the gas he had voluntarily inhaled.

Normally the muscle stiffening, rigor mortis, becomes obvious soon after death but the rate of onset, and that of the other natural physicochemical changes that occur in the body after death, are influenced by exogenous and endogenous factors. In the case of rigor, temperature is the most important factor, the ambient and body temperatures at the time of death. The temperatures in the UK and Ireland are moderate and in general the entire body will become rigid within twelve to twenty-four hours but this will gradually wear off and the body may become floppy twenty-four to forty-eight hours after death. In hot climates this is accelerated, the entire process over within a few hours, while in low temperatures, less than 10 degrees, the muscles may never stiffen.

The other changes we depend on are livor mortis and algor mortis. Livor mortis is more commonly called lividity, the reddening of the skin. This is due to the stagnant liquid blood in the vessels pooling under the effect of gravity; the uppermost surface of the body will be pale while the part of the body in contact with the ground will be red or purple. If the person is lying face up, the face will be pale, a comment often made by those who find a body: 'I knew he was dead because he looked so pale.' The blood takes some time to congeal after death, so if the body is moved, this will be reflected by a change in the pattern of lividity. After about twelve hours the blood will have congealed and a change of position will have no effect. This can assist in determining if a body was moved from one place to another, or its position changed, after death.

If the discovery of DNA was the 'eureka' moment for forensic scientists, the discovery of a logarithm that could calculate the time of death using the temperature of the body after death was lauded by forensic pathologists as the tool that would revolutionise murder investigations. Way back in the 1840s Professor Rainey had observed that the internal core temperature of a body drops after death, which he subsequently ascribed to Newton's Law of Cooling. The body was assumed to be roughly cylindrical in shape and therefore would cool at around the same rate as a cylinder.

Over the years further research was carried out in an effort to define the factors affecting the rate of cooling, in order that, by taking the body's temperature as soon as possible after it was found, the time of death could be calculated. Eventually the forensic pathology community accepted one logarithm but there was a large margin of error and many variables to take into consideration. Exact science it was not. Some pressed on with it, giving a definitive time of death to the team investigating, while many of us impressed on the police, in particular, that this should be regarded as a rough estimate. At times the best I could do was 'He probably died on Tuesday afternoon, rather than Wednesday.' I think that was very helpful, but the police were often dismayed: 'But, Doc, that means somebody else could have done it. Our man has an alibi for Tuesday afternoon!' Precisely!

In the last few years this evidence has been discredited in court. Most of us were right to be guarded about giving a definitive time of death. Professor Bernard Knight's adage has it that 'If you know when they were last seen alive and when were they found dead, they died sometime in between.' Wise words. When I'm teaching students, gardaí or anyone attending a crime scene about determining the time of death, I give them a simple rule of thumb: all anyone has to do is to try to move an arm and a leg, and feel how warm, or cold, the body is under its clothing. If the body is warm and floppy, the person died within the last couple of hours; if the arm and leg are stiffening but the body still feels warm they have been dead for a few hours; if the limbs are stiff and the body feels cold, death occurred twelve to twenty-four hours earlier. This is a very rough guide but, particularly when dealing with a potential murder, it assists the team investigating the death by giving them a time frame of when death occurred and therefore who could be responsible. Where were you between 8 and 10 p.m.? Where were you on Tuesday morning?

None of this corporal evidence was of any help in determining when our lady was murdered due to the time lapse between her death and her body being found. What else could be of assistance in narrowing down the time interval? Well, in these circumstances other environmental or associated evidence may be helpful. A newspaper may provide a day, a pile of post, evidence of a 'last' meal –

we're not proud. Any little clue might be helpful, even knowing a person's daily routine, anamnestic evidence. When did he last drop in for a paper and a packet of cigarettes on his way to get a bus? When did she last turn up for work? The police understand the importance of interviewing anyone the deceased would routinely come in contact with in order to set a time line.

A call came through to the police. An elderly woman was concerned: she hadn't heard from her sister for over a week, which was unusual. It transpired that every Tuesday night her sister would call her, and she had missed the call the night before. She rarely left the house and in twenty years had never missed a call. The police tried to establish how her sister had seemed when she last spoke to her: did she complain of feeling unwell or had she told her about any fall? The woman explained that she hadn't actually spoken to her sister for a long time, they hadn't much to say to each other, so why waste the price of a phone call? The routine was that she would phone her sister, let it ring three times, cut the call, and wait for her sister to call back, three rings and stop. If there was a problem they spoke to one another, even if it wasn't a Tuesday. She said she'd tried a few times that Tuesday night and now she was really worried. She lived in England and her sister was in Scotland and there was no way she could pop round. The police assured her that they would contact the relevant local police, who went to investigate, assuming the worst – she was in her eighties.

The police arrived to find the door of her flat unlocked. It was mid-morning but the curtains were drawn and the house was gloomy, but pristine. There was no evidence of any disturbance, but neither was there any evidence of the woman. The bedroom was tidy, clothes folded on a chair and the bed was made. Only when the curtains were thrown open and the room flooded with light did it become apparent that something or someone was under the covers of the bed. The bedspread was tentatively pulled back to reveal the missing sister. She was obviously dead, but she was lying face up, pillow over her face, her legs outstretched but her arms crossed over her chest, as if she had been laid out after death. While this was a shocking find, the next was even more so: in the corner of the room, initially hidden by the darkness, a figure was crouched.

The woman's son was crying quietly and it

was assumed that he was distraught at finding his mother dead, and had covered her body out of respect. By the time I arrived, he had been removed but one look at the old lady told me all I needed to know: she had been smothered. Another sad tale of family conflicts, a son driven to kill his mother. He was suffering from mental health issues and his marriage had broken down. Living with his mother, who was extremely demanding and particular about her house, was the last straw. Luckily the sisters' routine uncovered the crime, in more ways than one, sooner rather than later.

Unlike the elderly sisters, the young woman found strangled had no regular routine, her life was rather haphazard, but the police had one witness who was pretty sure she had seen the deceased on the high street eating a coconut iced bun, a Glasgow delicacy. This was the last known sighting.

Routinely, during the course of a postmortem, a sample of the stomach contents is retained if it is thought it might help with the time of death or piecing together last known movements, such as a visit to a burger van or a late-night kebab. On this occasion the stomach contents were fairly well digested and I wasn't confident of my ability to identify desiccated coconut. Time to look for an 'ologist, someone expert in identifying plants, fruits and vegetables. Not someone from the local garden centre, but a botanist.

At that time our office was deep in the bowels of Glasgow University, which was brimming with world-class experts. I checked the map of the university campus, and, jar in hand, set off to find someone in the botany department who would be willing to assist in a murder investigation. There is always someone, like myself, who is so intrigued by solving the puzzle that they don't think too much about consequences, in this case perhaps having to testify in a murder trial. I explained that a young woman's death was being treated as murder and the contents of her stomach might be of relevance in the investigation. What I omitted to mention was a coconut iced bun. I left the jar and waited.

A couple of days later I had a call: 'There was the usual mix of well-digested vegetable and meat cells, but one unusual finding was what appears to be coconut!' That's why I love an 'ologist. The eye-witness's account was corroborated, the time line was established, and now the police could do what they do best: find the perpetrator.

A plethora of 'ologists can contribute to a

forensic investigation. Sherlock Holmes said, 'You know my method. It is founded upon the observation of trifles', and now we have the science and technology to investigate the microscopic minutiae that will support our 'gut feelings', by providing pieces of the jigsaw that is the investigation of a murder. We have access to a variety of independent experts whose individual areas of expertise may provide the information that identifies a scene or a perpetrator: from pollen to foliage and body fluids to DNA analyses, there is an 'ologist who can help.

Of course, there is the collective group of crime-scene 'ologists, a mix of police and scientists, who are a constant in any investigation, my partners in crime. On a daily basis these forensic experts are called upon to provide assistance in investigating assaults, rapes, murders, drug-related offences, robberies, and more. In a murder investigation, a photographer, a fingerprint expert, a ballistics expert, a mapper and forensic scientists will be involved. The crime will dictate the forensic expert of most importance.

My greatest ally in a death investigation is the forensic photographer: they will provide the permanent record of the body at all stages of the examination. The photographs they take will be retained indefinitely; the better the photographer, the better the records. I have been extremely fortunate, particularly in Ireland, that all the garda photographers have been excellent. Nowadays as we have entered the digital era there is no limit on the number of photographs I can ask to be taken; previously I was dependent on the number of rolls of film that the photographer brought along. Sheepishly, some photographers would inform me before we started the postmortem that they had only one or two rolls of film with them. The silence that followed such a remark was usually sufficient for them to make a phone call back to the station for urgent supplies.

Although I take handwritten notes at all stages of my examination it is invaluable to have photographs to refer to. Being so close to the body as I examine it, the photographs afford me the opportunity to revisit it and to see it from a distance, which sometimes reveals more – injuries showing a distinctive pattern or a bruise that was not visible under the 'normal' lights of the postmortem room. It is a second chance to make sure nothing is overlooked.

While the individual forensic experts, particularly the forensic scientists, have a valuable contribution to make to the overall investigation, the bloodstain pattern analyst is most valuable to me. I am no stranger to bloody scenes and I can tell a 'hair wipe' from a 'cast off' pattern, but I find their contribution invaluable in deaths due to complex head injuries, bludgeoning deaths, the head having been struck by an object several times. From the number and size of the lacerations I can opine as to potential weapons, taking into consideration the damage to the skull. An object such as a hammer will produce a relatively small, but recognisable, injury, whereas a large object such as a rock may cause multiple irregular injuries; multiple overlapping blows from a hammer might produce a similar injury. Analysis of the blood-splatter pattern will identify the number of blows struck and, taking that information into consideration, I can give a better description of the potential weapon used. Synergy and collaboration are the key to making best use of the forensic experts. None of us should be working in isolation.

When it comes to trying to determine the time of death once the body has gone cold there is one 'ologist who can provide valuable evidence: the entomologist. How you can develop a passion for the study of insects is beyond me, but each to his own, and I'm more than happy to exploit that passion if it will assist in the investigation of a death.

In the UK and Ireland, within a short time of death, often minutes, flies are attracted to a body by the odour of death, the release of volatile components. It's a bit like the smell of bacon frying to us: instant salivation at the inherent promise of a tasty morsel, and gravitation towards the source. Can you blame a fly? We are rich pickings. The blow-fly, or bluebottle, may arrive within minutes and sets about laying eggs in cosy dark places, the eyes, nose and ears, and any orifice they can populate. The common housefly is not in such a hurry but waits until the putrefactive process is under way, possibly a couple of days. The eggs will hatch and the larvae, or maggots, feed on the body. There will usually be hundreds and thousands forming a swarm, moving *en masse* across and through the body, devouring any rotting tissue in their path. You can literally see steam rising off them, such is the ferocity of their activity.

The maggots grow until they reach a stage known as third instar. Then they are satiated and leave the body to find a nice safe place to pupate. This migration is important to the entomologist examining the scene, and why they prefer the body to be left in situ until they are certain they have all the evidence they need. Finding the pupa cases is the most difficult and time-consuming part of the scene examination, trying to predict where the larvae have gone and having to rip up carpets or dig deep into soil. This is often where amateur entomologists go wrong.

I am an amateur 'ologist of many disciplines, including entomology. I know my limitations and when a professional is required. For a start I don't really know one fly from another and I'm more intent at swatting them with a newspaper. Same goes for spiders. But that is key to the entomologist's calculations. Different flies have different life cycles and that is a crucial factor in determining when the fly laid eggs on the body: not the time of death, or postmortem interval, but the colonisation interval. Second, the growth of the larvae is dependent on the ambient temperature and its fluctuations so detailed meteorological charts for the period of interest have to be obtained and analysed.

It's not just a simple matter of arithmetic. I have had the joy of working with Dr John Manlove, a forensic scientist specialising in entomology. He has worked on several cases in Ireland, mainly in an effort to narrow down the postmortem interval. From the elderly lady who had been dead for months before her body was discovered, to the woman who had been murdered and her body dumped in a wooded area. Although entomologists prefer to see the body in situ, this is not always practical. But with modern technology I can be directed remotely, having had a crash course in collecting maggots and searching for pupae. The specimens can then be transported to the laboratory where the maggots will be reared under controlled conditions; this takes a few weeks.

This supposes that flies had access to the body from the time of death, but in winter months when the ambient temperature is low flies are relatively dormant and will not be active until the day heats up. Bodies are sometimes wrapped in plastic or other coverings and flies cannot get access; bodies are buried or even put into airtight containers such as freezers. These actions will obviously prevent flies getting immediate access to a body, which will affect the entomologist's calculations.

One interesting aspect of the fly's actions, from the pathologist's point of view, is that it will also lay eggs in wounds. This has implications for the living, as well as the dead. In cases of severe neglect, I have seen bed sores in the elderly infested by maggots. But this pattern of fly egg deposition has been helpful when the state of decomposition is such that it is difficult to be certain of the exact cause of death.

One young man went missing from a psychiatric unit. He had been admitted for treatment of depression. Despite a high level of security, he managed to slip out of the ward undetected. A full-scale search of the hospital and its grounds was carried out as soon as his absence came to the attention of the nursing staff, but to no avail. About ten days later a worker clearing the grounds of the school adjacent came across a body in an area of undergrowth. The police were alerted and immediately it was assumed that this was the missing patient. There was advanced decomposition of the body with maggot infestation. Fortunately, as part of the investigation of the missing patient, all records, including dental records, had been obtained, and this accelerated the positive identification of the young man. But how had he died? Apart from large collections of maggots on the face there were masses on both lower arms and on the neck. Flies had obviously been attracted to these areas of the body, the sites of predilection for self-inflicted injuries. This poor young man had deliberately left the security of the hospital to take his own life. The family was at least grateful that his body had been discovered and his fate was known. Death can be brutal.

Maggots feed on tissue and body fluids and therefore may sometimes be useful in certain deaths, notably those due to drugs. The feasting larvae will become intoxicated by any noxious substance that has been ingested or injected into the body. These drugs will also affect their lifecycle: for example, cocaine will speed it up. In cases where the extent of decomposition has destroyed the usual matrices for toxicological analyses – blood, liver or other body fluids and tissues – maggots can be used to determine the presence or absence of drugs that might have caused a death. Not favoured by toxicologists, but this is a last resort of the pathologist. In the few cases where I have found it necessary, the analyses have proved fruitful and a cause for the death has been found.

Toxicological analyses are routinely carried out during the investigation of a death if it is thought that alcohol or drugs were responsible for, or may have contributed to, the death. The toxicologists prepare and analyse samples of blood and urine.

Alcohol and drugs are commonly found, often together. Occasionally a death is due to consumption of alcohol alone, acute alcohol intoxication, but it is a common companion of deaths in violent circumstances: either the victim, the deceased, or the perpetrator may have been under the influence of alcohol at the time of the incident that led to a death. It is by no means an excuse for violent behaviour but I often comment that alcohol and certain drugs may have affected the actions and reactions of an individual, including not realising the potential danger in a situation or being reckless. Alcohol starts by freeing inhibitions, the giddy stage, but as levels in the blood rise it will depress the brain, the slurring and staggering stage, and if drinking continues the brainstem is affected, breathing slows and the conscious level drops, the comatose stage.

Certain drugs, heroin and tranquillisers, have a similar, and potentially lethal, effect with or without alcohol. Cocaine is another potentially lethal drug. There is a certain amount of snobbery in drug-taking, and probably to a certain extent in drinking. With alcohol, people buy what they can afford in the quantities required to attain a certain level of oblivion; just remember that Châteauneufdu-Pape is as lethal as Buckfast, even if you are drinking out of a crystal goblet rather than a bottle wrapped in a brown-paper bag.

With drugs, it is not the price that divides the 'rich' from the 'poor' but the drug itself. Alcohol has one effect, and people are of the opinion that the more they pay, the less the chance of noxious side-effects. Maybe just drink a bit less alcohol and more water. But drugs are a whole different ballgame. Oblivion versus high excitement; heroin and tranquillisers versus cocaine and ecstasy. Blot out life versus enhance life. Sorry, but you can still end up dead. Alcohol is regulated so the levels can be calculated: you know if you have more than four glasses of wine or you mix your drinks a hangover is inevitable. Unless the drugs you are taking are on prescription, buying from the guy hanging around the corner of the street or lurking in the dark recesses of a nightclub is the equivalent of playing Russian roulette – you pay your money and you take your chance. Good luck.

Cocaine came to our attention when it was discovered to be a common factor in deaths characterised by bizarre, paranoid and sometimes violent behaviour. The affected individual would be sweating due to hyperthermia, often throwing off clothing to cool down. This unusual behaviour obviously attracted the attention of the police or security personnel but the affected individual could not be calmed down and attempts to restrain them were almost impossible due to their apparent superhuman strength. This condition was identified as a state of excited delirium. Unfortunately attempts to restrain, on occasion, resulted in death. Death in these circumstances is worrying as it has occurred during attempts to arrest, a death in police custody. Preposterous: the people who should be keeping the peace and looking after us were causing the death of our citizens. Or were they?

These controversial deaths came under intense scrutiny. While cocaine was a common factor, it was realised that the pathophysiology of these deaths was far more complex than a simple 'bad' reaction to the drug, compounded by the rough handling of law enforcers. Sometimes the brain is just hanging on and a chemical reaction provoked by a drug might be sufficient to set off a cascade of reactions that might end in death. There is still much to be learned regarding these deaths and it is essential that police are trained in dealing with such fraught situations.

Nowadays toxicologists face a constant battle in keeping up with the drugs on the street. As do pathologists, if they cause death. One of the greatest challenges in recent years has been the influx of 'legal' highs, psychoactive drugs that were being peddled as safe party drugs. Unfortunately, there is no such thing as a safe drug: all drugs have side-effects, even the humble aspirin. These drugs were aimed at the young and, in the early days, were sufficiently under the radar that they could permeate the market. Fortunately, there have been few deaths, but sufficient to bring these drugs to the attention of the authorities. Legislation was introduced to limit exposure of the young to such potentially dangerous substances. The problem has been that the formulae are constantly being tweaked and this means that the toxicologists have to 'tweak' their analyses to make sure that any 'new' drug is picked up on routine testing before it causes a death.

Illicit drugs do not come with a list of potential side-effects. Neither are there warnings not to take them if you have mental health issues, not that those intent on taking illicit drugs are going to heed naysayers. Better not to take drugs that are not prescribed for you by a medical expert, but if you do and it goes wrong, I did warn you.

A fire broke out in a house in Galway at night. The fire brigade was called and attended. A couple of people had managed to get out. They had even tried to get back in to help others still inside but were beaten back by the flames and heat. Three bodies were removed from the smouldering building. Two had been in their thirties and one in her sixties. The male was found at the top of the stairs. The two females were found in their beds. It was assumed that they had all perished in the fire. The bodies were fairly badly burned but were still identifiable. The postmortems showed soot in their airways, confirming that they were alive when the fire started. Blood was sent to toxicology to quantify the level of carbon monoxide, the irrespirable product of combustion, which causes death by asphyxiation.

In the meantime, the other question to be answered was, why did they not escape the fire? The most obvious explanation is that they were rapidly overcome by the fumes. But people can be trapped, their path blocked by flames or falling masonry, or even immobilised by fear. Children are known to try to hide, under beds or in cupboards, rather than flee.

Smoke can also be disorienting, particularly if the victim is also confused by lack of oxygen. An elderly couple died in a house fire. They had lived in the bungalow most of their married life. The fire was due to an electrical fault. It started in the hall and spread to the living room and the bedrooms towards the back of the house. The couple were found dead in the living room. It would appear that they were awakened by the fire and made their way into the living room. As the smoke cleared, the walls told the story of their final minutes: handprints showed their frantic attempts to find a way out. How many times had they looked out the windows or walked through the doors? Blinding smoke, panic and lack of oxygen confused the situation and sealed their fate.

The Galway story was different. All three had high levels of carbon monoxide in their blood. But why did they not get out even when the alarm was raised? The male had recently broken his leg and was in a full leg plaster. He was trapped upstairs due to impaired mobility and was overcome by fumes, collapsing and dying, unable to get down the stairs. Toxicology provided the reasons why the two women had never stirred and died in their beds: one was intoxicated with alcohol and the other had taken a sleeping tablet; the pathologist and the toxicologist worked in concert to provide the families of the deceased with the full facts.

Positive toxicology might hold the key to the cause of death but, conversely, negative toxicology can also be helpful. Four women were found dead in their home. They kept to themselves and neighbours had not seen them for a week or so. The bodies were found by the landlord. The door was locked and barricaded. Finding four bodies is unusual, sufficiently so that the coroner, Professor Cusack, went to the scene to see for himself. I met him outside the house, and once photographs had been taken of the interior, we entered.

Inside there was an overwhelming stench of TCP, a smell I remembered from my teenage years and battles with acne. It was so powerful it almost, but not quite, masked the odours of putrefaction. The house was spotless and ordered. The only things out of place were the bodies of the women. The oldest was separate from the others, and our assumption was that she had died first and the others had laid her in the position she was found, almost as if she had died in her sleep, except she was not in a bed. In contrast, the other, younger, women appeared to have been left where they collapsed and died. There were no injuries apparent on any of the bodies. There was precious little food in the kitchen and no real evidence of food being prepared or eaten. The curtains were drawn and the house had a gloomy air.

When we opened the curtains, we were surprised to find that the windows were taped closed, ensuring no circulation of air into the house. Further exploration revealed that the fireplaces had been blocked off. There had been a deliberate attempt to make the house airtight. My immediate impression was that this had likely been a suicide pact and that death could have been due to suffocation from carbon dioxide or monoxide poisoning or that they had ingested a toxic substance. Either way, I was of a mind that, whatever had happened, no one else had been involved and that it was a joint enterprise.

I described the findings to the toxicologists and asked them to look for anything unusual that the group might have ingested and to check for carbon monoxide. Nothing unusual was found in any of the bodies. The postmortems showed some respiratory disease in the oldest woman, but no significant natural disease in the others, certainly nothing that could have caused their death. However, the three younger women showed features of terminal dehydration. There was no food in their stomachs and the small and large bowel were strangely empty. Gastroenteritis had to be excluded as a cause of general debility and death. There was no evidence of any infection or inflammation of the gastrointestinal tract or anywhere else in the body.

At the inquest, the coroner heard evidence that at least one of the women had been an advocate of fasting and had visited retreats especially for this purpose. By a process of elimination, the cause of death was determined at the inquest as dehydration and starvation, water deprivation being the major cause. The older woman, by virtue of her age and respiratory problems, probably succumbed several days before the others. An extraordinary collective decision. Who knows what goes on behind 'barricaded' doors?

People are sometimes confused about the distinction between the forensic pathologist and the forensic anthropologist. In simple terms the pathologist deals with bodies, flesh and blood, and the anthropologist deals with bare bones; the pathologist is medically trained, the anthropologist is a scientist; the pathologist deals with modern remains, while the anthropologist is generally more comfortable with old and ancient remains. But their spheres collide during the forensic investigation of deaths.

Over the years I have worked with some excellent anthropologists, Dame Sue Black in Scotland and Sierra Leone, and Laureen Buckley in Ireland, as well as the numerous anthropologists from America and England who were assisting the UN in the investigation of war crimes. Although their main role is identification of human remains, the American anthropologists, in particular, are also experts in bone injuries. I learned a lot about gunshot trauma to the bones, simple things like being able to determine the order of gunshots to the skull: the first shot causes a cobweb pattern of fractures radiating out from the hole punched by the bullet; this modifies the fractures caused by any subsequent shots as fracture lines do not cross a pre-existing fracture line, but come to an abrupt stop. A single shot to the head is usually sufficient to cause devastating injuries and death; with multiple shots, death is inevitable, but being able to give as much information as I can about the injuries adds to the overall picture of the incident. Every little helps!

Thanks to the anthropologists I can recognise animal bones, although some are trickier than others. The buried remains of a dead dog were thought by a local doctor possibly to be human remains. I had to trek over hills and down dales to the scene, where I was handed a spade and everyone took a step back. It took just a few scoops of earth to uncover the tail bones, definitely not human. And at the site of intended building work at the Red Cow in Dublin, the finding of a body turned out to be a pig. How a whole pig ended up buried was a conundrum. I needed Laureen for that case as initially only the 'chest' area was exposed and ribs can be a little difficult to identify.

Archaeologists are to be found at all building sites in Ireland, their role being to oversee the excavation phase, alert for any evidence of ancient settlements, and to prevent loss of valuable information that might throw light on the lives of our ancestors. They are interested in physical evidence, walls, buildings, roads and artefacts relating to how people lived, but occasionally they will come across human bones, bodies or apparent burial grounds. The builders have to down tools as human remains have to be reported to the coroner. What happens next depends on an assessment of the age of the bones: ancient versus modern. In general, there is a cut-off point of fifty to seventy years; even if it is suspected that the bones, or a body, might have belonged to someone who had met a violent death, there will not be a full investigation of the death as it is unlikely that the killer would still be alive.

The osteo-archaeologists on site are able to distinguish ancient from modern bones better than any doctor so I always respect their opinion as to whether or not I should deal with the find or the museum should be alerted. In Ireland in particular, there was rarely a week without bones, usually animal, or ancient remains being discovered. Very few required the attention of a forensic pathologist.

In 2003, a farmer cutting peat came across part of a body. The gardaí were alerted, the coroner contacted, and I was asked to attend at the scene in County Offaly. I arrived at about the same time as the Garda Technical Bureau: this was being treated as a potential murder. The body had been covered over with some plastic or a tarpaulin by the archaeologists. The photographer set about taking a series of photographs once it was uncovered. Then I was called over to make a preliminary examination.

To my amazement the 'body' comprised a torso and arms; the head and legs were missing. The skin was coppery brown and looked leathery. There was an amulet around one upper arm. This was my first bog body, Old Croghan Man. I had seen forensic pathologists give presentations about bodies possibly a hundred years old or more, preserved in ice or a bog, but I had never seen one in the 'well-preserved' flesh. Luckily an archaeologist had also been informed and I was given my first lesson on the power of the bog to preserve bodies.

This unique microclimate preserves and tans the skin, while bones are demineralised. I was astounded by this fine specimen. The physique was obviously that of a muscular man. As the arms were intact I could estimate from his span that he was about six feet. Once it was agreed that this was a bog body, I was no longer required. The museum were contacted and were delighted to receive such a fine specimen.

That should have been that. Some time later I was contacted by the museum: they wanted a multi-disciplinary team of experts to examine Old Croghan Man and would I be interested? Of course! What an opportunity. A team of experts from Ireland, the UK and Europe was amassed, all of us itching to get our hands on the body. I was there as a forensic pathologist to look for signs of trauma and to try to give some indication of how he had died. Samples had been sent for dating purposes so by this time we knew that he had died in the Iron Age, between 400 and 200 BC. Incredible. How fortunate was I that I was allowed to handle, with extreme care, such a valuable piece of Irish history? It soon became apparent that, while it could not be fully excluded that the damage to the body had been caused by peat-cutting machinery, he had been deliberately beheaded. There was also a stab wound to his chest, overlying the heart, which would almost certainly have been responsible for his death. Small samples were taken of internal tissues, and there was still recognisable lung tissue present. Radiology examinations were made and samples from the gastrointestinal tract examined to identify the diet of that time. I was honoured to have been involved.

Since then I have also examined Clonycavan Man, the upper half of another Iron Age bog body, with his distinctive elaborate hairstyle, and then in 2011 Cashel Man, who lived four thousand years ago in the early Bronze Age. Their stories are not for me to tell – the experts at the museum are far more able to do them justice. Tales of kings and kingdoms long forgotten, treachery, treason, torture and death. Oh, to have been a forensic pathologist in those days. I am thankful to the team that they allowed me to be a little part of rediscovering the history of our forefathers. Visit the bog bodies in the National Museum of Ireland in Dublin: they are magnificent.

Anthropologists and forensic pathologists are among a handful of 'ologists dealing with tangible evidence, something you can see, touch, feel and smell. Courts and juries can make up their own minds and accept or disregard our evidence and opinions. They have become amateur sleuths: thanks to *CSI*, everyone is an expert.

The other 'ologists are working in a world we cannot see so we are wholly dependent on that expert to describe their evidence, whether it is microscopic or the result of analyses carried out by machinery devised to detect and quantify certain substances, natural or unnatural, or sequences in DNA analyses. The evidence of these experts is ethereal. It is beyond our knowledge and we have to hope that there are sufficient checks and balances in place to ensure that it is reliable: calibrating the equipment used by toxicologists to measure levels of drugs and alcohol to ensure accuracy; peer review of microscopic slides and results of any scientific analyses. Check and check again. For several years now it has been mandatory that doctors have their reports and decisions peer-reviewed. This was routine in the Office of the State Pathologist long before it became compulsory. The forensic pathologist knows that every day the decisions they make could have adverse repercussions, suspicion falling on someone for causing a death, a murder missed, unnecessary upset to relatives. We have to get it right, if we can. Cases are discussed and dissected with colleagues, and if they cannot help, opinions will be sought further afield.

But what happens if someone manipulates or falsifies evidence, or deliberately, or unwittingly, misleads the courts? What if the 'ologist is of the opinion that the end justifies the means and their evidence is biased towards the prosecution or the defence? Or the 'ologist holds a belief that the evidence supports a theory not accepted by their peers but which they are convinced is true? Rogue 'ologist or misguided 'ologist? At some point someone came up with the crazy idea that the earth was spherical, not flat. A couple of thousand years later, with scientific and photographic proof of it, there are still 'flat earth believers'. What we believe to be true today we may have to reconsider tomorrow. And so it is with advances in science and medicine.

Even visible evidence can be manipulated by one side or the other in a murder trial. Forensic pathologists are of the Cinderella school of evidence: if the shoe fits the foot it could be a match but other feet might also fit. But imagine the scene in the court during the trial of O.J. Simpson for the murder of his wife and her friend when a glove was presented in evidence, a bloody glove found during searches of the scene of death and O.J. Simpson's house. All eyes are on O.J. as he pulls the glove down over his fingers. He struggles with it, his hand held aloft. He admits defeat: the glove doesn't fit; he's not 'Cinderella'. Despite his DNA and hairs being found at the murder scene, the jury acquitted him of both murders. The power of tangible evidence: they could see the glove, they could touch and smell the glove, and it was demonstrated that it did not fit. 'If it doesn't fit you must acquit.'

Sometimes experts hold beliefs contrary to accepted opinion. Only science can determine who is right and who is wrong. But sometimes the conflicting expert opinions may not be so divided but become polarised by the adversarial nature of the courts in the UK and Ireland. One opinion battles another when we should be striving to reach a level of agreement, then exploring our differences. The forensic pathologist called on behalf of the prosecution should explain to the court what their opinion is but also, as an unbiased expert, should also explain that there are contrary opinions and why they disagree with them. In general this leads to minor disagreements in court between the 'opposing' experts, rarely affecting the outcome of a trial. Pathologists do not hold the power.

However, when the deceased is a baby, and there is evidence to suggest that its death was due to inflicted trauma, there is likely to be a battle between the prosecution and the defence. All of the evidence will be questioned, and the pathologists and 'ologists have to be prepared for a gruelling time in the witness box. This is not the usual dilemma of intent to injure, manslaughter versus murder: this is the fundamental question of whether or not the trauma was the result of an accident or was deliberately inflicted. Accident or murder. This is a fight for justice for a child who has suffered at the hands of another versus a fight for justice for a person wrongly accused of harming a child. Strong stuff. Both sides must have evidence to support their claims and that evidence must withstand the rigours of court.

The experts called upon by the prosecution have to remember that they are experts for the court and not the prosecution: it is not for them to prove the case for the prosecution. It is essential that the expert is aware of current theories and research in the field and whether or not it supports their opinion. It is important that the expert is not entrenched in their beliefs and is willing to consider alternative theories and opinions, whether or not they agree with them. I have tried to follow that path throughout my career. Whether or not I succeeded is for others to judge.

These cases would not have reached court if the prosecution thought there was insufficient evidence to support a charge of murder. It is for the defence to rebut that evidence. They must show that there is an alternative explanation. In baby cases this means presenting evidence to show that the injuries purported to have been inflicted could have occurred accidentally. The defence will look for an expert who will give an alternative, or directly opposing, opinion to the one presented by the prosecution.

One of the most controversial diagnoses is that of shaken baby syndrome: a child has been shaken with such force that it suffers brain injury and dies. Much research has been carried out and there are conflicting theories of how the brain injury is caused, ranging from the believers in shaking, to those who argue that there must have been more than shaking, to those who dismiss trauma as the cause of the brain injury and offer other 'natural' causes. Wide-ranging opinions all needing to be addressed and assessed.

Non-accidental injury, causing death, usually, but not always, because of head trauma is another controversial diagnosis. Is there an innocent explanation for the trauma? At trial the defence will attempt to undermine the case for the prosecution and the pathologist's evidence by calling an expert who has opposing views to the prosecution case.

Sadly, I have had to deal with several babies who have died from head injuries, which were suspected to have been caused deliberately. In each case I expected my evidence to be challenged. Naively, when I first became a forensic pathologist,

I believed everything I was told and trusted that everyone was being truthful. As the years went by, and the murders I dealt with multiplied, I realised that life is not black and white and neither is the investigation of murder. I have never set out to mislead the court but I realise now that I might have put my trust in assertions made by those I assumed to be older and wiser. Medicine is not an exact science, and now we are focused on practising evidence-based medicine. We don't follow blindly without questioning. A welcome step forward. It has become apparent that we are still a long way off understanding and explaining some of our findings. Once you accept that what we earlier believed was not necessarily correct, it is easier to be objective and unbiased, and not dismiss 'new' science as hocus-pocus.

It is probably easier for me than the other members of the team investigating a suspicious death to accept that there are other possible explanations for the pathological findings and therefor manner of death. I have no axe to grind, no personal hypothesis to defend. On the contrary, I am more than willing to accept a novel theory if there is scientific evidence to back it up. We are constantly pushing the boundaries of medicine and science, and we should embrace the progression of knowledge: advances in science and medicine are only achieved by challenging current theories, which might be hypotheses in disguise.

As a scientist I like to be able to solve a problem step by step, proving the validity of each along the way to the solution, or the hypothesis never attains the level of a 'theory' or a 'law'. A question mark remains. That was the state of forensic pathology when I began but, over the years, sterling work has been done that has brought a greater understanding of many diseases and, for the forensic pathologist, a clearer explanation for death in some circumstances.

It is easy to dismiss as a charlatan someone who questions your opinion and has a diametrically opposite opinion, but that is counter-productive and not helpful to the court. Experts are chosen by the defence team because their opinion may be beneficial to their client's case. It is for the court to decide which opinion, or what evidence, supports or refutes the prosecution case. As baby murders are relatively uncommon and the pool of experts is small, the same experts crop up time and time again. Forensic pathologists most commonly give evidence for the prosecution in these cases, as they have carried out the postmortem on the child, but often experts from other branches of medicine will be called upon by the prosecution and the defence. Some of these experts are called upon exclusively by the defence because they have a controversial viewpoint, contrary to opinions held by their peers. Unfortunately, this may earn them a reputation for being pro-defence and not impartial. It is for the judge to decide who should be regarded as an expert in a trial and therefore whether or not that person may give evidence. Forensic pathologists are generally regarded as experts but some have fallen foul of the court system and have been discredited.

In the course of my career I have met many who challenged my opinions but only a few whose motives were questioned. One was a biochemist with an interest in bones and the other a paediatric neuropathologist with an interest in shaken baby syndrome. Our paths crossed because babies had died in seemingly violent circumstances and the parents or carers were being accused of their murders. Both of these doctors were admirable in attempting to find an explanation, or at least an alternative explanation, for injuries in children where the only evidence of deliberate harm was the presence of an injury or a pattern of injuries that was said to be diagnostic of deliberately inflicted trauma, the so-called non-accidental injury.

I have always been wary of such provocative terminology: it implies that a decision has been made regarding the circumstances before a full investigation has been carried out. I don't use the term 'non-accidental injury' to describe a head injury in an adult, even when there is clear evidence to suggest that it was deliberately inflicted: why should I use such an inflammatory descriptive term when describing a head injury in a child? 'Deliberately inflicted trauma' may be top of my list of differential diagnoses but I must remember that there may be another explanation. Of course, when considering the explanations given to account for any injury, I take everything into consideration – relationship to other injuries, pattern – as well as all other postmortem findings; a wide-angled view, rather than fixating on one particular injury.

This was where the two experts and I differed in our approaches. Their opinions were based on only one aspect: the biochemist on the broken bones and the neuropathologist on the changes in the brain. They did not take into consideration the other findings, which supported the possibility that those children could have been murdered. I would argue that they were right to limit themselves to their specific area of expertise. But were those limitations made clear to the court in view of the opinions they expressed?

While the biochemist was an expert in bone metabolism, he was not an expert in child deaths or paediatric pathology, and he should have made that clear to the court. In contrast, the expert paediatric neuropathologist questioned the validity of the diagnosis of 'shaken baby syndrome' and appeared in court several times to present her alternative point of view.

Pathologists recognised a pattern of trauma in babies, consisting of subdural haemorrhage, brain injury and retinal haemorrhage, known as the 'triad', which they thought could be caused by vigorous shaking of the child, and that was the accepted belief for many years. However, recent thinking has questioned it. Much research has been carried out by well-qualified experts in mechanical engineering as to whether shaking a child could generate sufficient force to cause such significant trauma to its brain; some say no, some say yes.

In addition, research by neuropathologists suggested other possible explanations for the brain trauma that had originally been attributed to shaking. It was proffered that it was possible that the changes to the eye and brain could be due to hypoxia, lack of oxygen, which caused the brain to swell and the pressure inside the skull to rise, not necessarily due to trauma, shaking in particular. But how to prove or disprove these hypotheses? There is still limited, or insufficient, scientific evidence to fully support them. Despite that, the impression given to the court by this expert for the defence was that research had proven that shaken baby syndrome was no longer a valid diagnosis. Shaking did not create sufficient force to cause the brain injury and there was an alternative explanation for it. There was no evidence that the child had been deliberately injured.

The problem for the courts is that they are very dependent on the pathologists' findings as, generally, the events leading to the child's fatal brain injury are not witnessed by an independent party. What a dilemma for the court. Two opposing opinions. The fact that there was some doubt as to whether or not shaking a child could cause such severe injury to the brain was sufficient to raise doubt in some courts, much to the annoyance of some forensic pathologists.

This paediatric neuropathologist quite rightly questioned long-held beliefs about brain injury. If there is some scientific evidence to support alternative theories, they cannot be dismissed. We just need more research to clarify the situation. However, she should have explained that she was not a forensic pathologist, and that her opinions were based solely on the findings in the brain and did not take into account any other injuries, not even fractures of the skull.

It is essential that all 'ology experts realise the limits of their expertise. Those who make extraordinary claims must provide extraordinary proof in support. But also, when speaking out against mainstream views, you must acknowledge the limits of your knowledge and not express opinions on matters outside your area of expertise.

It is inherent in us to try to be helpful – do charity work, help old ladies across the road, have a bake sale to raise funds for the local school. Just do not fall into the trap of being cajoled into answering any question if this is not within your area of expertise. If pressed to answer, or you feel compelled to answer, always qualify your answer with the statement 'This is not my area of expertise'. It is also important that if asked by the prosecution or the defence to give an opinion in any case, do not assume you were the expert they really wanted: you may be the sixth person they asked. Other, more experienced, experts may have declined, often because they are too busy. Sometimes they decline because they would rather not get involved in the case.

If you agree to get involved, always make sure you know what you're being asked to opine on and ask yourself if you are the 'expert' with the correct expertise for this particular case. Don't be the 'expert' who is known for appearing as the generic expert witness, the Jack or Jill of all trades. In many cases, having read the evidence available, I often explain that the expert they need is not me and point them towards someone else. Sometimes I wish the defence the best of luck – the evidence suggests they're going to need it.

It is essential to avoid a miscarriage of justice. 'Convicted by juries, exonerated by science': we must ensure that the jury's decision in any case is based on the sound, solid scientific evidence of all 'ologists, including myself. Never assume that because we are scientists our evidence is necessarily correct. None of us is infallible.

10

The Other Side of the Tape

FOR MORE THAN THIRTY YEARS I have spent my time telling the stories of the dead. I have been their voice. I have seen death in all its guises: the gentle and sometimes beautiful natural end to a life well lived and its opposite. Sometimes death can be brutal in its suddenness, the killer showing a callous indifference to our life expectation. The only thing for sure is that life will end, one day.

While I am more aware of that than most, I do not fear death: it is the few minutes before that are more of a worry. What happens after, to your soul, your essence or your energy? Who knows?

In my career I have met remarkable people: the

stoic relatives who bear the most awful tragedies with grace; the fearless families who will take on a government to get changes in the law; the professionals who care, including the police and the gardaí, as well as APTs and undertakers; the forensic experts who never cease to amaze me with their brilliance.

If there have been changes in forensic pathology over that time, they have been subtle. But it is wonderful now to look around at a conference and not be the only woman in the room.

Doctors shy away from death but we, the pathologists, have always tried to make some sense of it. Only by determining how and why people are dying can we hope to prevent further deaths in similar circumstances, be that natural disease, death due to drugs, road traffic incidents, suicides and even homicides. Funding can be directed into research, drug centres, counselling services, and into personnel to keep us safe. We should never underestimate our contribution to life through our work with the dead.

Life is short and that seems to be on people's minds quite a lot these days. We have entered the era of the bucket list. No longer is it sufficient to tell anyone who wants to listen, or even cares, that you are thinking about a fancy five-star holiday. No, every proposed trip is now qualified as 'It's on my bucket list.' Really? If you want to go on safari, see the Northern Lights, surf off the Maldives, or whatever, save up, drop into the travel agent or book online. We don't care. Why should I feel inadequate about preferring a week in Blackpool to a week in Bali?

And as for 'experiences', bungee-jumping off the Golden Gate Bridge, swimming with sharks, are you off your head? That is a guaranteed bucket list, a 'death wish' list. Show your videos to someone who cares. Does anyone?

If you want to do something useful, look after people, even those you don't know, listen to them: you may be very interesting but others are too in their own way – and, above all, be kind.

And so, for the last time I put the scalpel down, pull off my apron and gown, scrunch them into a ball and slam them into the bin. I pick up my notes, the door of the mortuary swings open and I take one last look to make sure I haven't forgotten anything before the door closes with a thud behind me. Wellies are discarded – the name on the side will fade in time – and other feet will take them back into the mortuary. I push open the door to the corridor and the art deco staircase sweeps up and around in front of me. I climb the stairs that separate the dead below from the living above. The sound of my heels on the marble echoes through the stairwell, heralding my imminent arrival.

The gardaí are huddled around the table in the tea room, mugs and empty sandwich wrappers strewn in front of them. Their voices still and they look up expectantly. 'It's a murder. Just give me a minute to grab a cup of coffee and I'll fill you in on the details.'

For one last time I tell them a story, the unique and special story of how the person lying on the mortuary table below met their death.

For the first time I'm on the other side of the tape with you, a bystander looking in. Over there is the Technical Bureau's van: it must be serious. Look, there's the photographer. That's probably the state pathologist. Can't really tell in those awful white suits. I wonder what happened, who's dead? How did they die? If only I could duck under the tape, what a tale they would tell me.

Acknowledgements

I would like to thank everyone at Hachette Ireland for your perseverance in getting me to this point, especially Ciara Considine. I knew I would be in safe hands from our first meeting. This would not have come about if it was not for my agent Faith O'Grady, who has guided me through the unfamiliar world of publishing and the media.

There are so many people who have influenced me along the way. I am grateful to those who said 'No' to me in my early career, my life could have been very different. More important are those who supported me: Rod Burnett who let me get my foot in the door of pathology – those were very happy days in Stobhill Hospital; John Clarke, on whom I was foisted, sorry I was so annoying; Jack

Harbison, an incredible character who brought me to Ireland, and Bernard Knight who championed me at my interview, the forensic pathologist I most aspired to be.

Everyone I have worked with in Glasgow and Dublin has been a joy, well that might be a slight exaggeration, but I've met more good people than bad. Thank you. My last twenty years in Ireland were great, mainly because of the people, especially the Garda Technical Bureau, the State Laboratory and Forensic Science Ireland, as well as the APTs in all the mortuaries in Ireland. Of course, I could not have been the state pathologist without all at the Office of the State Pathologist, particularly the three musketeers, Ciaran, Daphne and Lorraine, in alphabetical order, not in order of importance. You are all important to me. Over the years my forensic families became my friends.

To my family: Phil, who had to function as a single parent a lot of the time, and my fabulous children Kieran and Sarah. I did miss you when I wasn't there but at least you knew I would be coming back to you, although it was touch and go in Sierra Leone. Not forgetting Monica, my little sister who always looked up to me, mostly because she's two inches shorter.